THE FORGOTTEN REVOLUTION

THE PRIORY METHOD

A RESTORATIVE CARE MODEL
FOR OLDER PERSONS

JESSIE MANTLE & JEANETTE FUNKE-FURBER
IN DIALOGUE WITH VERA MCIVER

Printed in Victoria, Canada

Book design, Roy Diment, VRG
www.members.shaw.ca/vrg

National Library of Canada Cataloguing in Publication

Mantle, Jessie, 1932-
        The forgotten revolution : the priory method :
a restorative care model for older persons /
Jessie Mantle, Jeanette Funke-Furber ; interviewee, Vera McIver.
Co-published by: Greater Victoria Elder Care Foundation.
Includes bibliographical references.
ISBN 1-55395-749-0
        1. Aged--Institutional care. 2. Aged--Rehabilitation.
3. Aged--Medical care. 4. McIver, Vera--Interviews.
I. Funke-Furber, Jeanette, 1942- II. McIver, Vera
III. Greater Victoria Elder Care Foundation IV. Title.
V. Title: The priory method.
RC954.3.M36 2003   362.6'1   C2003-900813-4

TRAFFORD

This book was published *on-demand* in cooperation with Trafford Publishing.
On-demand publishing is a unique process and service of making a book available for retail sale to the public taking advantage of on-demand manufacturing and Internet marketing. **On-demand publishing** includes promotions, retail sales, manufacturing, order fulfilment, accounting and collecting royalties on behalf of the author.

Suite 6E, 2333 Government St., Victoria, B.C. V8T 4P4, CANADA
Phone   250-383-6864   Toll-free   1-888-232-4444 (Canada & US)
Fax   250-383-6804   E-mail   sales@trafford.com
Web site   www.trafford.com   TRAFFORD PUBLISHING IS A DIVISION OF TRAFFORD HOLDINGS LTD.
Trafford Catalogue #03-0112   www.trafford.com/robots/03-0112.html

10   9   8   7   6   5   4   3   2

Contents

List of Figures and Tables

Acknowledgements

The material in this monograph is drawn from a variety of sources. The majority of the material comes from discussions with Vera McIver herself, augmented by her unpublished manuscript written in 1999. The material is drawn from these two sources unless noted otherwise and is not footnoted to facilitate ease of reading. In addition we had available to us written copies of her conference presentations and teaching notes, as well as her published writings. The works of other authors writing in the field of long-term care, both published and unpublished, are used to enhance the material where necessary. Two films made available to us by the former Juan de Fuca Hospital Society provided us with the living record captured on film. [1,2]

Our work was greatly advanced by the reviewers of our manuscript. Carolyn Attridge, Mary Buzzell, Lucia Gamroth, Marian McGee, Janice Robinson, Meryn Stuart, and Fiona Sudbury gave their time and their wise advice to help us with this task. Maureen Cranwell, who worked with us as Executive Secretary during our active careers, provided editorial and secretarial assistance with the commitment to quality that she always manifested. Our Social Work colleague Dorothy Wing, now also retired, modified the original drawings of the Tree which was the first metaphor which McIver developed to portray Restorative Care.

Finally, a big thanks to the Greater Victoria Eldercare Foundation (formerly the Juan de Fuca Hospital Foundation) for their generous grant which brought this important history to print.

[1] National Film Board of Canada. (Producer). (1979). The Priory: The Only Home I've Got. Ottawa, Ont.

[2] McIver, V. (Producer). (1968). The Priory Method - Extended Care - Remotivation. Videotape made from a 16 mm Movie Film. Juan de Fuca Hospitals, Victoria, BC.

Dedication

We would like to dedicate this book to Gladys Lofts RN, with whom we worked at Juan de Fuca Hospitals. It was she who brought the writings of Vera McIver to our attention and who told us about the Priory Method. She had worked with Vera for many years on the Priory site. Just before she died we were able to visit her in hospital and we told her we were writing this work. Her eyes lit up with excitement to think that the ideas of the Priory Method would now be in print. That light has been our inspiration.

Preface

In Charles Dickens' *A Christmas Carol*, written back in 1843, two business men seek a donation from Scrooge to assist the poor. Scrooge refuses and claims he supports the workhouses and that is where the poor should go. The businessmen are appropriately appalled and indicate that the workhouses are dreadful and, in fact, some poor people would rather die than go there. Fast forward to 1967 to Victoria, B.C. and view The Priory through Vera McIver's eyes: monotonous environment, only superficial attention to the medical needs of the residents, no rehabilitation, excessive use of restraints both chemical and physical, no activities or social stimulation, no warmth and personal involvement between nursing staff and residents. It is likely that many old people would rather have died than go there. In fact, there is not that much difference between these two "houses" once the civilizing effects of the intervening 144 years are taken into account. Neither type of establishment had any recognition that a home is more than the provision of food and protection from the elements. Neither took responsibility for ensuring that people lived their lives to the fullest rather than put in time until death. Add another 36 years and in 2003, the need to create a real home for functionally dependent and cognitively impaired older people is still only slowly being recognized across the long term care community, i.e., a home that includes privacy, interpersonal warmth and commitment between residents and staff, an interesting and stimulating environment, opportunities for continued personal development and for contributing to others, encouragement to use ones' abilities to their maximum, and assistance to live life as fully as possible.

How did Vera McIver get so far ahead of the rest of the field? She had picked (or more accurately had it thrust upon her) an area of health care that had little prestige and few resources. There were essentially no role models for her to follow. Furthermore, she brought a background in acute care nursing, exactly the kind of background that had helped to create the sterile, excessively routinized environments she found. Yet, she was not trapped by that background, as were her contemporaries both within and beyond nursing. Somehow, she was able to translate her ideas of how to bring life and living to the Priory into a set of principles that could be generalized so others could also follow them. This was theory based nursing before the term was invented. Even more impressive, she developed a set of management principles so that the practice change could be implemented across the Priory and other organizations.

The Priory Restorative Care Model contains most elements now recognized as essential to a progressive residential environment for older people. For example, the visiting hours were eliminated. Visiting hours are an institutional concept, not one associated with home, where coming and going, sometimes expected and sometimes not, are the norm. In several areas the Priory Method continues to be ahead of the field at large. For example, true interdisciplinarity including role overlap, was the norm. Staff members used their professional expertise and their personal skills to make the Priory a community that was lived by all, not just the residents. Housekeepers led hymn singing, cooks danced with residents, and secretaries played the piano. Contributing to life was everyone's responsibility, not just the activity coordinator's. Physiotherapists taught the nurses and health care assistants to carry out the rehabilitation routines residents required, rather than insisting on doing them all by herself which would have led to fewer sessions for each person. The multiples roles in providing care were assumed by whomever possessed the skill, not just the professional designation. Overcoming disciplinary boundaries and territoriality may be the most difficult hurdle in creating a community that has the objective of being responsive to the needs of individuals who live and work in it.

Vera McIver not only developed theory to guide practice, she used administrative theory, a rare occurrence in the health care environment of the 1970's. The management theorists of the time, Hertzberg, Likert and Argyris, provided her with principles and approaches of working with professional and non-professional staff that were congruent with the way she wanted them to work with and be with the residents. She freed the staff from the tyranny of a hierarchical management structure to participate in a more complex but more flexible one that included multiple reporting relationships. This type of structure requires an organization with great trust in its employees because they are telling different people different things about what they are doing and no one is responsible to insure they are doing it all.

Vera McIver attributes her passion for long term care and her creative ability to the Holy Spirit. That may have been her source of inspiration but she was able to translate this passion to a human level so others who may not have had the same spiritual inspiration could be inspired by her. She worked in very human ways and made it possible for others to exhibit the same levels of commitment that she had to the residents they were entrusted with.

This book on the Priory Method by Jessie Mantle and Jeanette Funke-Furber is a most important contribution to the history of long term care and nursing in long term care in Canada. It clearly acknowledges Vera McIver as the source of the creative ideas behind the Priory Method. What Jessie Mantle and Jeanette Funke-Furber do not take credit for is insuring that the Priory Method survived and thrived after Vera McIver was no longer available to shepherd it on a day-today basis. The Juan de Fuca Hospitals had a reputation for being progressive and for incorporating new practices and roles ahead of other long term care facilities. Jessie Mantle, one of Canada's most creative nurses in the field of gerontology, was one of the early clinical nurse specialists in a long-term care setting in Canada when she joined the Juan de Fuca Hospitals. Jeanette Funke-Furber maintained the administrative innovation and energy in the 1980's and 90's that Vera McIver brought two decades earlier. Their commitment to maintain and build on what had been established was crucial to allow the Priory Method to flourish. There is only one task left to do: reinstate the name "Priory Method" and recognize it as incorporating a distinct and logical set of principles and practices.

Dorothy Pringle RN PhD
Professor & Dean Emeritus
Faculty of Nursing, University of Toronto
January, 2003.

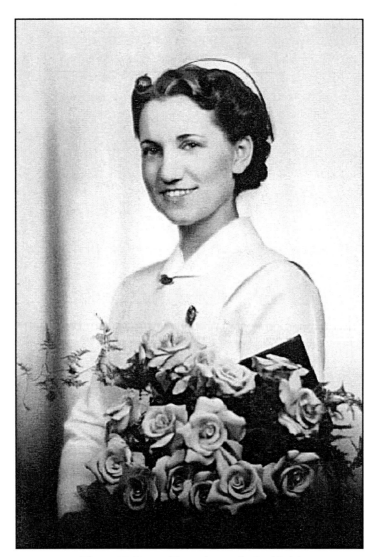

Vera McIver (Dombowsky) 1941
Regina Grey Nuns Hospital

Notes by Vera McIver

I always had a strong calling to be a nurse. Even as a child I made it known to the family that I was going to be a nurse and the desire never left me. I enjoyed my nurse's training and career. However in 1967, when Sister Mary Elizabeth OSB, my sister, in charge at St. Mary's Priory asked me to move to Victoria to be the Nursing Director of their extended care unit, I was reluctant. I was too steeped in the prevailing false impression that working with the elderly wasn't challenging. In all honesty, it was beneath the dignity of a <u>good</u> nurse! But to please Sister I said I would accept for six months, just long enough to introduce a programme for the newly established extended care unit. It wasn't nepotism; Sister could find no one else. When the six months were over, I was hooked; I had no intention of leaving these wonderful old folks.

A transformation took place in my psyche as I began working at the St. Mary's Priory. I saw needless degradation and knew changes had to be made to enrich the lives of these unfortunate patients. I kept striving for excellence, not only in efficiency and economy but also in improvements to the patient's environment and daily living experiences. This feeling was so profound I simply had to express it. Before this time, I had neither written nor lectured on any topic. Now, I would do either at the drop of a hat. I could not stop myself. I truly did not know where my energy and abilities to do this came from. I seemed to have unbelievable stamina and capacity to work. Latent forces and talents must have come to the fore as my consciousness expanded and I came alive with this new endeavor.

Since I was directly responsible for all the care provided by all the disciplines and services, I studied and read by the hour, critically analyzing the material with a discerning mind as to it's application to the programme of care, which became know as the Priory Method. I was open to change. I wasn't attached to any one programme or model of care. I had always worked as a private nurse, working in many settings but always directly for and with the patient.

Often, completely unrelated articles would trigger a beneficial insight or inspiration. The nursing and medical literature at the time had little to offer in caring for the elderly so I studied psychology and sociology and even went further afield. Often, ordinary magazines offered helpful materials, e.g. I read an article on the ecology of the forest and the forestry practices that were causing devastation to the forests. I applied this to the environment in long-term care facilities. I realized that we had devastating practices for the patients who lived in these facilities and what we were doing in the environment could be detrimental to the life of patients.

I also read about the brainwashing techniques used by the Koreans on the American prisoners' of war. To have their captives be subjected to the most severe experiences, the soldiers' rooms were stark with only a cot for furniture and a single light hanging from the centre of the ceiling, which was left on 24-hours a day. I looked at our patients' rooms and we had all these conditions. That's when I began realizing that we had to change. We began with splashing colour on the walls and beds. We personalized the residents' living space around their bed, with their own possessions and mementos in the hope that this new ambience would assist in the remotivation programme we were developing for the residents.

I saw resistance and resentment from some sources who did not approve of the change. A non-committal role was easier for some of them. I did not let this deter me; I knew we had to go forward. It was as if a cell in my brain was set free and channeled my creative thoughts in one direction. I set weekly and monthly goals, always striving to improve towards excellence. I was single minded. I was consumed by a passion to bring humanity to all those who became my responsibility. As Wayne Dyer a noted American TV lecturer of Wisdom of the Ages says "the music must come out!"

I thoroughly enjoyed my work; it was too enjoyable to feel like work. My enthusiasm bubbled over to those around me, which helped them enjoy their work. Staff was able to maintain a cheerful and positive attitude in spite of the fact that they were caring for mentally and physically disabled individuals. Anton Karch M.Sc., University of Calgary was able to attest to this during his research at the Priory.

I could not understand my total conversion and passion for long-term care. My late 98-year-old sister, Sr. Mary Elizabeth knew exactly where it came from, the Holy Spirit! To be a part of the lives of the residents as they improved with the new programme was very rewarding; "they are like trees that grow beside a stream, that bear fruit at the right time and whose leaves do not dry up." (Good News Bible, Psalm 1 Verse 3)

Vera McIver August 2002

Introduction

The purpose of this monograph is to describe the characteristics of and the developmental process used to create the Priory Method – a care system for the institutionalized elderly developed at St Mary's Priory in Victoria, British Columbia, Canada. Although the model was developed over thirty years ago, it has a contemporary ring to those who continue in this sector of health care. By putting this information into the public domain we hope that readers will be informed about the salient features of the model and may be inspired to incorporate aspects of the model in their current practice settings. As we go to press the health care system is once again in crisis and advances made in the past are at risk of being lost. The shift to a preoccupation with health care costs is challenging some of the innovative ideas found expressed in this book. Yet again there is a need for creative and informed leadership if the rights of residents for humane and quality care are to be preserved.

We hope that readers from all walks of health care will be excited by this example of improving care through innovation and commitment. It illustrates how one person might seize opportunities for change provided one has the courage and vision to do so. Vera McIver, a registered nurse at St Mary's Priory, began developing the Priory Method of helping the elderly in 1967 when she became Director of Nursing. At that time the facility was owned and operated by the Sisters of the Love of Jesus who followed the Benedictine Rule. The name 'Priory' has a Christian origin and refers to a religious house. The nuns provided extended care nursing to 95 resident older women. When the Priory Method was developed, it challenged the prevailing approach of custodial care or what Baum has called "warehousing the elderly."[3] The method was aimed at treating seniors as normal people rather than as sick patients. The Priory Method enabled the residents to regain many abilities that had been lost by the dependency forced on them in the sick role. Many of these individuals came to participate as functioning individuals in their "home" and in the surrounding community challenging the stereotypical images of nursing home patients as no longer of value to society. Over the years Vera McIver and the Priory Method became known not only throughout Canada and the United States but also in England, Germany, Czechoslovakia, Israel, Jerusalem and Japan. McIver was honored for her work by a number of groups and was awarded the Order of Canada in 1986 and the Queen's Golden Jubilee Medal in 2002.

---

[3] Baum, D.J. (1977). Warehouses for Death: The Nursing Home Industry. Ontario: Burns & MacEachern Limited. ix.

We are privileged to document this work during a period of time when Vera McIver is still a healthy and vigorous senior living in our community of Victoria, B.C. Through our interactions with her we were able to capture her memories and her thoughts about what she had done, as well as why she had done things the way she did. This offered a rare opportunity to talk directly to someone who had created her work over thirty years ago rather than trying to work solely from published information and secondary sources. She had in her possession and made available to us copies of many of the original documents (hospital manuals, newsletters, letters, photographs, newspaper clippings and papers) which reflected the development of the Priory Method.

Throughout the preparation of this monograph we were struck over and over again by the creative spirit of Vera. She brought in innovations and approaches long before we began our work in long-term care and which we thought were new in our time, albeit called by other names. Working in the late sixties and early seventies she was formulating and using ideas that only later came to be widely understood. Today her ideas are commonplace and words such as Restorative Care, multi-tasking, hospice care for the severely demented and holistic care emanating from these ideas are better understood and accepted by practitioners in all walks of health care. But in her time and in her work setting of institutional care for the elderly, her ideas were novel to most and understood by few.

How did one person swim against the tide of the time and find the vision that would change health care for the frail and ill-institutionalized elderly? An examination of McIver's past sheds some light on this question. Vera McIver had always been an entrepreneur, learning new concepts and studying wherever her need for knowledge led her. She had a deeply held philosophical belief system derived from her Roman Catholic faith and this was reinforced in her basic nursing education at the Regina Grey Nuns' Hospital in Saskatchewan. She graduated from her nursing school in 1941 and rather than practice as a staff nurse in the acute care hospital, she chose to become a special duty nurse. These nurses were usually associated with a Private Duty Registry rather than a hospital. When a hospitalized patient needed more nursing care than the assigned staff could provide, the Registry would be contacted and one or more nurses would be assigned for the duration of the required intensive care. The usual practice was that patients paid for this service. In this role, McIver was able to focus her whole attention on an individual patient and his/her nursing needs. This experience formed her strong belief that all quality care must be based in a patient-centered approach made manifest at every level of an organization. Nothing else was more important to her than the patient as a person.

By her own admission her major strength lay in the fact that when she began at the Priory in 1967 at fifty years of age, she was mature and financially independent. This enabled her to take risks and challenge the status quo. Her years of experience in nursing and in living had given her a sound basic knowledge. It also equipped her with a style of learning based on her innate curiosity that would lead her into new avenues of thought. Because of her financial picture she would not suffer an economic crisis if a disapproving board or manager threatened her job status. Thus she set forth on what was the greatest adventure of her nursing life. (McIver, V. 2001. Personal Communication)

The authors of this monograph were privileged to inherit the legacy of working with the Priory Method long after its development. During the 1980's and 1990's they were both in positions of leadership at the Juan de Fuca Hospitals, hospitals which included the original St Mary's Priory. The model had infiltrated throughout the organization although it was no longer referred to as "The Priory Method." So successful was the infusion of the ideas that the care practices derived from the model were largely taken for granted by all the staff as the way one provides care. It was only when one attended conferences that one realized that this was not the prevailing pattern in many organizations and that the quality of care offered at Juan de Fuca Hospitals achieved a very high standard. The source of the ideas and the writings about it were largely unknown by the majority of the staff, including the authors. We decided to write this monograph in the hopes of correcting this deficit for ourselves and for others as well as to pay tribute to the model's originator.

The authors have faced a difficult challenge in writing about these ideas. This model was an early example of what is known today as holistic care. By its very definition, holistic care does not break things down into component parts but rather integrates ideas of the person in his/her environment. It doesn't slice an individual into aspects such as physical, emotional and spiritual or cut an organization into departments or programmes. One is always working with an intact complete picture. Finding a way to portray 'holism' is not easy in a world where breakdown and classification are the order of the day. It needs the language of poetry, metaphor and/or artistic representation. McIver managed to find words, which were novel and more encompassing than the traditional language of health care practice and administration, but even she was unable to discover words that preserved an integrated picture of the whole. She did however use the metaphor of a tree to convey the interdependence of the elements of the lived experience of an institutionalized elder and we have included the tree metaphor in the text to convey this sense of holism.

This monograph covers the period of growth from 1967 when McIver was hired until 1979 when she retired. This is the period in which the publicly acclaimed Priory Method took hold as a driving force influencing the long-term care institutional programmes in Canada and beyond. What has happened to this model of care in to-day's practices? Unfortunately the model still remains unknown to many working in long term care. In other instances, the model has appropriately changed and evolved over time as the ideas have permeated the culture of long-term care.This is the case of the new facility, Heritage Woods, built on the old Priory site in 1998. In this facility a new generation of leaders in long-term care created an innovative model that reflects the seeds planted so long ago by McIver.A discussion of this model is found in the concluding chapter of this monograph.

In the chapters that follow we have tried to remain true to the vision held by McIver. She has said to us over and over that she was not a scholar but rather someone who saw that things just had to change and set about doing that. Her language was simple but eloquent, and it was the language of her day, not ours. For instance, words that describe power struggles and political activism come much later in the history of long-term care nursing and we had to fight the desire to use today's language in portraying her actions. She did not use words such as 'personhood' and we have resisted the wish to do so even though the spirit of her work suggests she would have much sympathy with this notion. We have followed her use of the terms of physiological, psychological, social and spiritual to describe the components of a human being rather than use our own frameworks even though the reader might be jarred by words which are no longer in favor.We have tried to speak with her voice to a new audience in a new generation of people concerned with how we care for older people.

Her ideas were developed intuitively and not from any pre determined plan or nursing framework. This left us with a problem about how to order the material because she did not develop this model in a time-sequenced systematic way. For ease of reading we have reverted to a sequential model acknowledging the evolution when we could. We begin in Chapter 1 with a description of the characteristics of institutional care for the elderly at the Priory as she began her work.The description of the Priory Method is found in Chapter 2, 3 and 4. Chapter 2 describes the beginnings of the model including the philosophy. Chapter 3 outlines the significant features of the clinical practice of Restorative Care and Chapter 4 describes the management environment she saw as essential to support that practice.While we have separated these for purposes of clarity, the reader should understand that these areas were so interdependent in McIver's mind that they cannot be separated in reality. She held a unique position – that of the clinical nurse leader *and* the manager of all the services involved in resident care.Any particular innovation that she made most likely simultaneously involved both practice and management changes.As we reflected on her position we could see the great advantage of this dual role for anyone who attempts change of the magnitude which McIver pioneered. Finally in Chapter 5 we look at how the model influenced those both within and beyond the Priory walls during the years of McIver's tenure and after her retirement. We invite the reader to journey back in time with us and enter the mind and spirit of a nurse who dared to think outside the box of traditional care for the elderly and change the world forever.

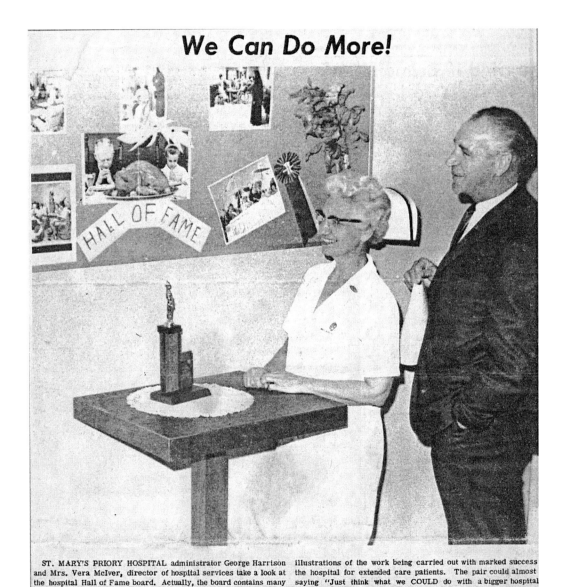

We Can Do More!

ST. MARY'S PRIORY HOSPITAL administrator George Harrison and Mrs. Vera McIver, director of hospital services take a look at the hospital Hall of Fame board. Actually, the board contains many illustrations of the work being carried out with marked success the hospital for extended care patients. The pair could almost saying "Just think what we COULD do with a bigger hospital

Juan de Fuca News Review. October 16, 1968, Colwood, B.C.

chapter 1

The Way It Was at The Priory
Pre 1967

The Priory Hospital existed within the context of the Canadian health care system as it related to long-term care for older people. It was this context that influenced the way older people were cared for. The patient profile was common to all like facilities. The staff and the care model reflected the prevailing paradigm of the day. It was her introduction to this paradigm that shocked McIver and planted the seeds for change that were to follow as she gained experience in the field.

THE CANADIAN CONTEXT

Institutional care specifically designed for elderly citizens is a relatively new phenomenon in the western world. In Canada, as in other countries, the elderly were considered no different than the poor and sick of all ages. The arrangements that developed to assist them varied by province. In its early days, this welfare was provided by "private and church philanthropy but the nineteenth century saw the gradual involvement of government bodies through legislation, financial support and inspection."[4] Forbes et al, report that in 1941 there were two hundred and fifty eight charitable and benevolent institutions across the country that housed 11,358 older adults.[5] More than half of these adults were 70 years or older. As the authors note, these institutions "provided custodial care to dependent and handicapped people…"[6] The elderly were also found in acute care hospitals and in convalescent and chronic care units or facilities but there were often insufficient beds and the services frequently lacked a geriatric focus. Institutional long-term care experienced a growth spurt after the Second World War when there was an increase in the number of elderly in the population as well as increased government financial incentives.

---

[4]   Forbes, W. F., Jackson, J. F., & Kraus, A. S. (1987). Institutionalization of the Elderly in Canada. Toronto: Butterworths. 14.

[5]   Forbes et al. 9-10.

[6]   Forbes et al. 9.

In the main, the first homes for seniors were remodeled buildings, operated by enterprising but inexperienced persons who were ready to fill a much-needed gap. When new homes or private hospitals were built, well-intentioned acute care oriented planners in government tended to plan for long-term care patients as they did for those in hospitals who were cared for in bed. In their minds these patients would be using bedpans and would be bathed from a hand basin thus leading to an insufficient number of toilets and bathing facilities for a resident population. The consequent reduction in usual mobility led to a loss of function in patients' muscles and bones. Patients would be eating their meals off trays in their beds rather than in a dining room as one normally does and activity areas were merely waiting rooms limiting what one could do in rehabilitation and recreation.

Forbes and his colleagues identified a persistent negative attitude towards institutional care for the elderly. In the eighteenth and nineteenth centuries it was believed that those in need of assistance were largely to blame for their situation.[7] The idea that it was their own actions and lifestyle that had necessitated their institutionalization, was a good example of 'blaming the victims' for their situation. This led to the acceptance of the custodial approach for those so blamed. This view was reflected in the attitude of potential residents. There was a stigma attached to being admitted to a Home. The phrase "put away" was used and old people were embarrassed to be admitted. Adult children were reluctant to push their parents out of their nest and into this unforgiving setting.

In his writings, Baum captures the mood and the approach in use at the time McIver began her work in long-term care:

> With few exceptions, … Canadians have placed increasing numbers [of elders] in nursing homes, homes for the aged and charitable institutions caring for the elderly. People are there to die. Once they walk through the nursing home door and take their rooms, they will not walk out again. They are stripped of their assets, given a small personal allowance, promised minimal nursing care, regulated severely in their routine and medicated to institutional compliance. In a very real sense, they are encapsulated and warehoused for death. They are removed from the community, and the community accordingly does not have to see either old age or death.[8]

---

7   Forbes, W. F., Jackson, J. F., & Kraus, A. S. (1987). <u>Institutionalization of the Elderly in Canada</u>. Toronto: Butterworths. 15.

8   Baum, D.J. (1977). <u>Warehouses for Death: The Nursing Home Industry</u>. Ontario: Burns & MacEachern Limited. 3.

THE HISTORICAL ROOTS OF ST MARY'S PRIORY

The Priory Method developed within an organization that was already focused on the needs of older people. In 1951 after many other entrepreneurial endeavors, Mother Cecelia, founder of the Sisters of the Love of Jesus, purchased a site in Langford, near Victoria. It was bought from the Royal Colwood Golf Club and consisted of a large clubhouse, the Chez Marcel Restaurant, the caretaker's house and other smaller buildings on nine acres.

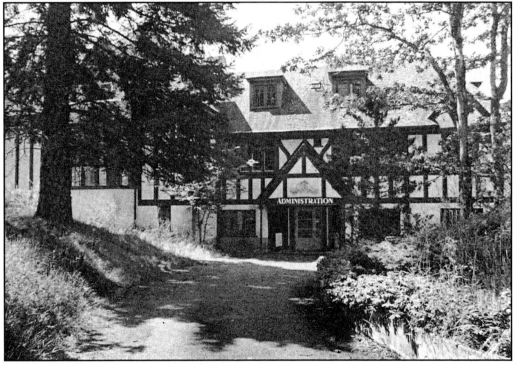

St. Mary's Priory Hospital

The clubhouse was renovated to serve as a convent for the Sisters as well as accommodation for 48 patients, and was named the 'Priory Convalescent Home'. In fact the patients here were the severely mentally impaired elderly. Over time, Mother Cecelia created a setting that allowed for the development of a full range of care for about 200 older people (predominantly women). The caretaker's house was converted to a Medical, Dental and X-ray centre. A commercial laundry and a maintenance shop were established in the garage. In 1953 the restaurant was converted into a 24-bed hospital and was named 'The Little Hospital'. This never was a hospital as such, but a care facility. In 1955 Mother

Cecilia built the House of Peace, according to her own plans. She hired a local builder who used day laborers. It was to house 91 patients but with over-crowding it often housed closer to 100 elderly people. In 1957, Mother Cecelia bought the property across the street, the Royal Auto Court, and converted it into a house for well seniors in retirement. (Dombowsky, Sister Mary Elizabeth, 2001, Personal Conversation)

The finances that Mother Cecelia provided for the operation of the whole complex with its full range of services were meager for meeting even the basic needs of the elderly. In addition, she had become engrossed with the care of dogs, animals that she loved. The dog issue grew out of control and when Mother was ordered by the Department of Health and Welfare to get rid of the dogs, she chose to leave the site. Thus in 1962 she lost control of the operation of the Sisters of the Love of Jesus. With her departure The Priory operation had little cash flow and the books were in the red. The remaining Nuns and the staff of nurses and aides continued on caring for the older people in the typical manner of the times.

In 1966 an advisory board was formed to assist the Sisters in their financial dilemma. The British Columbia Hospital Insurance System (*BCHIS*) agreed to take over the 24-bed hospital as an extended care unit for which they would pay the operating expenses. On February 1, 1967 the House of Peace (which became the Priory hospital) was also accepted as an extended care unit with the proviso that the patient count be reduced from 91 to 71 residents and that necessary renovations be made. Renovations were undertaken both for the House of Peace and for the Little Hospital and resulted in the provision of extended care services for 95 residents.

The advisory board recommended that an administrator and a nursing director be hired. On April 1, 1967, George Harrison who had been working for BCHIS was ready for a change and assumed the position as administrator. On June 1, 1967 Vera McIver, in an unusual move given her past experiences, took over the nursing director position and began learning about how to care for long-term care patients. Here we see the first glimpse of the McIver who was ready to break the mold of traditional practices in administration. She wanted firsthand information and she obtained this by going, herself, to the wards and working with the patients alongside the direct care staff. This is an approach that would be considered highly unusual then and now. But this approach proved very useful for it was from this experience that she identified the characteristics of the residents, the profile of the staff and the features of the custodial approach that she set out to change.

THE RESIDENTS

In 1967 the criteria for admission to an extended care facility required that potential residents have stabilized chronic diseases or functional disabilities, requiring 24-hour nursing care with professional medical and nursing services. At the operational level, the criteria for admission to an extended care facility were usually based on several factors either singly or in combination. The most important factor was that a person was unable to ambulate or operate a wheel-chair safely. Other criteria that were considered included:

Unable to get in and out of bed safely,
Require assistance in activities of daily living,
Require special diets,
Unable to self-administer prescription drugs,
Require services for physiotherapy and occupational therapy,
Suffer from mental confusion but not violent behaviour.

The patients, as they were called at that time, were all female and most of them suffered some degree of mental and/or physical impairment. They lived either in one of the four large 13-bed wards or in one of the 2-bed rooms. Most of them were bed-ridden and had very little contact with the outside world.

THE STAFF

The in-house staff was comprised of registered nurses and care aides supported by staff working in housekeeping, maintenance and the kitchen. Drug supplies came from an outside local pharmacy that charged a dispensing fee for prescriptions. There were no social workers, physiotherapists or nutritionists available to residents and their families.

The Health Care Team was comprised not only of nursing staff but also of physicians. While there was a house doctor who visited regularly, the patients could retain their own physicians. The medical staff rarely provided an adequate medical diagnosis. Most of the residents were diagnosed as being senile – a word that had very little meaning and which was often applied without any rigorous medical work-up. Drugs were similarly prescribed when residents had problems and often led to iatrogenic effects that worsened the problems they were trying to treat. The input of the physicians into care was minimal and they were rarely on site.

During her early work with the residents and the staff, McIver developed strong views about nurses. In one public seminar presentation she stated:

> Nursing [has] tended to become a mechanical function... She [the nurse] observes psychosocial concerns as a non-nursing function and resents the involvement. She wants to nurse, she says, but her actions belie her words.

She busies herself with tasks such as staffing, housekeeping, requisitioning and answering telephones. She "over-nurses" the chart with meaningless entries. It is extremely difficult for some to change from former established hospital attitudes, policies and procedures…Consequently, when the nurse is introduced to a people-oriented environment and she is stripped of many non-nursing functions, she lacks confidence and knowledge. She has not been adequately prepared to deal with emotional, social and rehabilitative problems. Her limitations and her resistance to the new work environment contribute to poor morale as her attitudes and conflict become apparent to the lower echelon.[9]

The causes of these staff behaviors were multiple and complex. The society in which the staff lived and worked devalued the elderly, especially those who were ill and frail. This had two effects. Firstly, many of these care providers brought these broader negative social values into their work environment and this affected how they behaved towards the older residents. Secondly, because of their affiliation with this work, health care colleagues in other fields devalued these nurses and aides thus affecting their self-image.

For the most part neither the professional nor the non-professional staff had any special preparation in understanding normal aging and illness in the elderly. The majority of the non-professional staff had no formal training in caregiving at all, but rather they had learned on the job and were strongly influenced by the environment in which they worked. Caring for seniors was a new career path for doctors and nurses. When McIver took over as Director in 1967 neither BCHIS nor the Canadian Hospital Association (CHA) offered any courses to train staff in long-term care facilities. In North America, geriatrics was not believed to be as challenging as work in a general hospital. Recruiting talented and educated staff to these facilities was and remains today, one of the major challenges.

The professional staff, predominantly registered nurses (R.N's), had received their education within an acute care hospital model and brought this experience to bear on their practices in long-term care. Their orientation was towards cure, an unachievable goal with chronically ill, aged persons.[10] They were at a loss as to how to set realistic goals for this population and how to reorient their practice away from the hospital-based acute care model. They spent much of their time following protocols from their acute care practice. For instance they routinely took the temperature and blood pressure of the residents who did

---

[9]   McIver, V. (1973, February 26). A new environment for extended care. Proceedings of the Seminar on Extended Care. British Columbia Hospital Association. Richmond, BC. 33-34.
[10]   McIver, V. (1972, January 19). Focus On Aging. Notes for a paper presentation at the Interprofessional Course. University of British Columbia, Vancouver, BC.

not display any symptoms necessitating these measures. Furthermore acutely ill, hospitalized patients have relatively short-term stays and are discharged to their home environments. Thus while the nurses were skilled in forming brief, meaningful relationships with patients they had little experience in creating on-going long-term relationships.[11]

All of these factors presented nurses with new demands on their nursing abilities for which they were unprepared. For instance when McIver was beginning the introduction of the Priory Method, an R.N was asked to reactivate a person's walking skills. The nurse was heard to say, "I did not go in training to walk patients," reflecting a complete lack of understanding about the nursing needs of the elderly. Sadly, as McIver noted, she probably didn't go into training to do inventories and other non-nursing duties either yet now these were prized activities and consumed a large amount of her nursing time. McIver argued that long-term care suffered because the majority of highly educated and dedicated nurses saw no meaning or value in this field and therefore it lacked leadership.

THE CUSTODIAL CARE MODEL

Nurses and doctors working in these environments thought that emulating the acute care hospital model could attain excellence.[12] This thought was challenged by relatively few. The care of the physical body received preference over the care of the person. The yardstick for the measurement of good care was the absence of bedsores accomplished through good "body" care. Staff expected patients to endure a period of dependency and being "looked after" although in this instance it was to continue for the rest of their lives. If the patient was too active, she or he was tranquilized. If this did not settle the person the dose of the medication was increased. In many cases physical restraints were ordered and applied. As McIver noted, when the patient was finally subdued-vegetated and no longer asking for anything, she/he was considered a "good patient". Patients were not exercised and diversional activities were rare. Soon patients were incontinent because of their immobility and in many cases a catheter was used on an on-going basis to maintain dryness. In the health care field this was the type of care giving that came to be known as custodial care.

With few exceptions, rehabilitation was not even contemplated. Illness and signs and symptoms were the preoccupation of the staff. Issues of personhood and family support that was of critical importance to the patients were never discussed. While custodial care based on the acute care model provided basic

---

[11] Mantle, J. (1994). Unpublished teaching notes. University of Victoria. Victoria, BC.
[12] McIver, V. (1971, August 19). <u>Acute Care Philosophy Versus Extended Care Philosophy</u>. Notes for a speech presented at Malaspina College. Nanaimo, BC.

physical care, it neglected some of the most important aspects of a human being's needs, namely, spiritual and psychosocial. McIver believed that when these patient needs went unfulfilled, the person lost heart and began to deteriorate.

The model of custodial care was supported by the staff's perception that they lacked time for care. The low budgetary allocations for staff provided by government funding agencies reflected the general view that long-term care patients did not require as much assistance as their counterparts in the acute care hospitals. This led to low staff/high patient load ratios and created a heavy workload. Staff believed that this did not permit time for more than basic care. McIver believed they did not use their time effectively.

The nurse and the nursing aide had to complete their workload during their shift so they could not allow for too many interruptions from patients. Patients were tied to their chairs because they believed they could come to harm if they were not under the nurse's watchful eye. Pleas to go to the bathroom were often ignored and incontinence became a way of life. A person who ate slowly was often prescribed a minced or blenderized diet and in order to save time the nurse often resorted to feeding the patient. In some instances even syringes were used to feed patients. Allowing the patients to dress themselves took time and so the care aide would take over this task further reducing the patients' skills and increasing their sense of inadequacy.

What seemed to be timesaving measures were double edged swords. Incontinence increased the risk of pressure sores and demanded increased hours spent in treatment. The inactivity robbed the muscles and bones of their strength and a patient who could have been walked to the bathroom at one time, now might have to be lifted by two nurses and taken by wheelchair. Minced and pureed diets led to loss of appetite and pleasure in eating and time had to be taken to coax people to eat with "please take another bite."

McIver describes the end result of custodial care as a cascade of effects set in motion. Physical health was compromised to the degree that a complete loss of mobility was the usual state of most patients. With only minimal social, emotional and spiritual attention being provided, the condition of many of the patients further deteriorated. Deterioration created increased dependency. Dependency killed the patients' sense of identity thus robbing them of their pride and dignity. With the loss of pride and dignity came mental deterioration and death of the human spirit. It was these observations that planted the seeds for change. Finding a way to reverse these changes became her task as she entered into her new role as Director of Nursing.

PROVINCE, Tuesday, February 27, 1973   ★★★31

Hospital walls 'should be ripped down'

By JOHN BRADDOCK
Province Medical Reporter

Institutions providing long-term treatment to the elderly or disabled will have to carry their work into the community, speakers said Monday at the B.C. Hospitals Association's seminar on extended care.

Inside the hospitals, they said, greater emphasis should be placed on personal care rather than administrative convenience.

Dr. Carl Eisdorfer, chairman of the psychiatry department of the University of Washington and former director of the Centre for the Study of Aging and Human Development at Duke University, said: "We should, metaphorically, tear down the walls" of hospitals. In the few cases where this has been done in the U.S. there has been "staggering success," Eisdorfer said.

Eisdorfer told delegates to to the two-day conference in Richmond that deterioration illness and senility in the elderly are not inevitable and, contrary to common opinion, it is possible to teach the aged new methods of adjustment. Even the so-called vegetative state can be reversed, he said.

He suggested extended care institutions should be "environmentally based with outreach programs" to prepare people who have to come in for treatment, but also help them later when they want to make it on their own.

Eisdorfer criticized situations in which an elderly person who is ill either has to go to an acute care hospital where the patient is diagnosed, treated and discharged as quickly as possible because of the expense, or goes to an extended-care unit—"a vegetable-bin business to keep them off the streets." Often an elderly person is physically ill but diagnosed psychotic and is treated with drugs without any attempt to determine the physical cause, he said.

Miss G. T. Alfano, director of Loeb Centre for Nursing, Montefiore Hospital, New York, said more time must be spent by the staff of extended care hospitals in discovering the needs of their patients. She said too often the institutions are run for the convenience of the administrators and janitors. Miss Alfano said nurses must assume the leading role in providing the new emphasis, and more responsibility must be given to the patient in assisting with his care.

The Province, Dec 3, 1971, Vancouver, B.C.

Woman's Province

A miracle from great expectations

First in

a three-part series

by Kay Alsop

THE OLD VEGETATE FROM 'SOCIAL AMPUTATION'

VICTORIA — Lights flick off in Vera McIver's small office. A projector whirrs. On the wall opposite figures flicker into action. A woman comes into focus.

Old, she is. Pathetic, her face creased with pain and a terrible sadness. Her eyes are dull, sunken. Her lips fold in on toothless gums. In the wheelchair, her body slumps, partly blanket-covered.

"She's in the process of dying," explains Vera McIver, over the whirr of the projector.

As director of services at St. Mary's Priory Hospital, Victoria, she knows, and tells, how the woman's well-meaning relatives deposited her at the hospital along with the medical verdict that she had only a short time to live.

While she's talking the film continues to reel off shots of activity in the hospital corridors, nurses, patients, chatting with a lovely lady in a mink jacket who, smiling and gracious, moves briskly from one person to another.

"It's the same lady," says Vera McIver quietly. "Six months later."

A moment of shocked disbelief. It CAN'T be the same lady.

The film is reversed, run through again, and still the change is almost impossible to accept.

The film clips along to show another miracle; a woman who sits hopelessly and mindlessly clenching and unclenching her fists, unable to get herself in or out of bed without the aid of two nurses. A few feet of film and the same woman is shown laughing

handing out a different kind of role.

St. Mary's Priory, operated by the Benedictine Sisters in Victoria, was one of the first nursing homes to be accepted as an extended care hospital, back in December, 1965.

In April, 1967, George Harrison, formerly assistant administrator of a 1500 bed hospital in Edmonton, took over as full-time administrator of the Priory. His enthusiasm for suggested innovations in programming has been invaluable, according to Mrs. McIver. He is credited, too, in the accreditation awarded the hospital in November, for "the organized manner in which he has developed this hospital," for his "interest, judgment, and an awareness of the needs of this kind of patient."

"Nurses talk a lot about Loeb Centre in New York, a most progressive centre but we have something equal in Canada and we find it at the Priory."

It's called The Priory Method. What it is, roughly, is a recognition of personality and the maintaining of human dignity, in people receiving extended care, a kind of Great Expectations.

"There's a great misconception about aging," says Vera

That same year Vera McIver, who had retired from active nursing, moved to Victoria with her husband, intending to just take it easy, maybe raise quarter horses or something to pass the time. Members of her family lived in Victoria, one of whom was

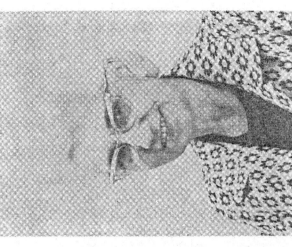

Vera McIver ... director of hospital services.

chapter 2

The Priory Model of Restorative Care
– A New Vision

Mcclver's brief period of evaluation in her new job led her to a passionate commitment to change the custodial care system. She was to call her approach 'Restorative Care', which she defined as a programme to restore dignity of life to older institutionalized persons within the limits of their capabilities. She saw this as an alternative to the vigorous physical rehabilitation programmes that were available for younger persons but which she thought were inappropriate for the capabilities of her institutionalized older adults.

In this chapter we deal with the intuitive development of Restorative Care. The basic components emerged out of McIver's interpretations of staff experiences with residents as they experimented with new care practices. They reflect the creative spirit in action rather than coming as a result of any pre-planned detailed design. The metaphor of a tree as a teaching tool came as an unintended consequence of a picture-taking project designed for another purpose. The philosophy driving McIver was consciously articulated only when a staff nurse urged that this be done.

AN IDEA IS BORN

How did McIver begin her approach to change the way patients were cared for? The vision did not come all at once and as she describes it, the model emerged slowly over time. She recalled:

> In hindsight one has to give credit to serendipity (a gift of being able to make delightful discoveries by pure accident). When we started the program in June 1967 we began by meeting our patients' basic human needs. It was so simple; it did not require any great imagination or increase in budget. We merely began by introducing them back to walking and simple exercises, [taking them] to the dining room and for bathroom privileges. We planned social activities in house and out to the community. Our patients (ladies initially) could not be seen in the hospital nighties with company coming to visit. Dresses and shoes were now a part of the daytime attire. Hairdos and perms were next. Make up and costume jewelry were the finishing touches to have them look gorgeous again. Can you imagine what

this did to their pride and self worth? Then purses were resurrected as they were in control of their own spending money. Living in these long-term care facilities they had been stripped of these essential day-to-day normal life activities. The result of all this new pride was a desire for more socializing and the staff also enjoyed this more normal ambiance and morale was high. (McIver, V. 2001. Personal Interview)

In 1967 McIver's somewhat unorthodox approach took her far beyond the traditional medical and nursing literature, which she found inadequately addressed the care of the elderly. She read widely and saw, for instance, how the social and psychological disciplines shed light on understanding the human organism and the relationship to space. Their literature on territoriality suggested ways to alleviate the stress and deterioration that could occur to people who are institutionalized in confined spaces. Broadening their horizons reduced the older persons' need to covet their own little space. In her view the buildings and policies had to counteract these tendencies and thus the notions of communal dining, indoor and outdoor recreational areas, and community outings and functions were given birth.[13]

Another serendipitous finding occurred when the activity coordinator, using an 8mm-movie camera, took pictures at all the festive occasions and a number of other events showing resident and staff activities. They would show the films to the residents as a recreational activity and they observed that this provided ego-enhancing experiences. As residents were seeing themselves in the movies they grew more aware of themselves and began asking for things like new clothes and hairdos. Their life was really becoming more worthwhile. After a few months McIver and the staff realized they had before and after movie segments in which the remarkable recovery of some of the residents was made visible. What they saw was a transformation that was hard to believe. It became quite evident that they had film of residents in severe depression and immobility to begin with and that a few months later, these same residents were bowling, were up in wheelchairs and visiting with children. McIver pieced these before and after segments together and realized she had the makings of an educational film. These pieces had to be organized into meaningful headings. Since there was no sound on the film, McIver created headings as a way of giving commentary to the film clips. These headings became the basic ideas of the model: messages of wellness; strengthening the body; strengthening the ego; humanizing the living space; and creating community.

[13]   McIver, V. (1973, February 26). A new environment for extended care. Proceedings of the Seminar on Extended Care. British Columbia Hospital Association. Richmond, BC. 36.

Daily Colonist, Victoria, B.C., Tuesday, July 8, 1959

18

Elderly Enjoy New Life
Thanks to Good Citizen

The Native Sons of B.C., Greater Victoria branch, conferred their 25th good citizenship award on Mrs. Vera McIver in Beacon Hill Park Sunday afternoon.

And after the ceremony there was a tea party at the Gold Cup. Among the many noticed were former award winners, Mrs. Ada Barner, Mrs. E. E. Harper, Mrs. Marjoie Naysmith, Mrs. Annie McVie, Harold B. Elworthy, Freeman King and Sgt. Roy Woolsey.

Each one of these names represents a singular achievement in connection with the welfare of this area.

Mrs. McIver, latest award winner, services director at

St. Mary's Priory, has introduced an entire new concept in the care of the aged in the short two years since taking over the post.

Of course, she is thrilled about the award, mainly because it gives recognition of a change in the nursing care for the aged that has been instituted with such overwhelming success at the priory.

★ ★ ★

The new comprehensive care, with stress on the social needs of the elderly, is in complete opposition to the old "bottom of the barrel" and "go to sleep" idea.

It takes an optimistic and positive approach rather than

just good care, says Mrs. McIver.

Mrs. McIver, a graduate of Greys Hospital in Regina, has many years of nursing service to her credit but actually came out of retirement to take over her job at the priory. And looked upon it as a challenge.

A challenge that has been well met judging by the results with the elderly patients.

Mrs. McIver had been interested in nursing care of the aged and has read quite a lot about a new approach to the care of the elderly.

She quoted from an article by Dr. M Oberleder, chief psychologist of the Geriatric Service at the Bronx State

Hospital, that what has formerly been accepted as brain damage was often "a reality denial defence or ego defence delusion and that senility is a systematic defence reaction." Also that memory loss, delusion and incontinence was curable, or at least could be ameliorated.

★ ★ ★

Mrs. McIver has given lectures and written many articles on the subject of the remotivation program for the aged.

The aims of the remotivation program are to encourage and develop our residents to the highest optimum level in personal adjustment, social

interaction and in leading a productive role," she said.

"Many of our patients have had tremendous trauma physically and mentally. It must be remembered that the average age at the priory is 83 years. Old age brings with it many infirmities and disabilities, as well as loss of family and friends."

As she says, lonliness, bitterness and despair set in and create a rejection and escapism until individuals withdraw into a protective shell and finally step into a world of fantasy that releases them from their self-imposed prisons.

★ ★ ★

Victoria Times, January 14, 1975.

HOME MOVIES BECOME REAL THING

A Time to Rejoin the Living

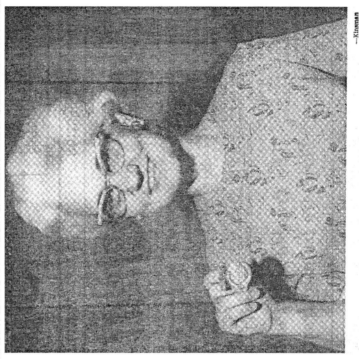

—Kinsman

Mrs. McIvor takes optimistic approach

Mrs. Nellie Allison assembles bonnets for African children

Differences

"Philosophis, attitudes and environment differ greatly. In the acute hospital, the patient is disrobed and clad in night attire to play the sick role. The aged person is viewed as a pesky problem . . . .

"At the Priory, pride in self is encouraged, the person is dressed in becoming attire and she is expected to pay the well role. We assume all have a potential for some recovery, we build on strengths.

"Our gains vary from a sweet smile to independence and we delight in both."

The nurse, says Mrs. McIver, must be concerned with the enrichment of human life, just as much as she is saving it. All the pills in the world won't bring back self esteem, ease grief, fear or guilt in an old woman. Nursing can.

THE METAPHOR OF THE TREE

As an aid to her thinking and teaching, McIver developed the metaphor of a tree. She visualized the *patient* receiving custodial care as a tree, starved for the nutrients needed to maintain identity as a human being. Only the physiological roots were being nourished by the most basic measures of nutrition, body care, medical treatments and drugs. The psychological and social roots went unfed. Spiritual needs were not addressed. Rather than generating strong branches and healthy leaves, this tree was withered and dying as a result of the complications bred by the starvation. The enforced immobility led to complete dependence. The physiological complications of osteoporosis, muscle atrophy, sensory-motor deprivation and other sequelae such as constipation and pressure sores abounded. McIver differentiated between psychological and social, eschewing the common practice of using the term psychosocial. She felt you lost information if you combined these words and while they were interrelated, they were also separate areas that must be addressed. By neglecting the psychological and social needs of the older persons, there was a loss of identity and social and psychological death. The psychological complications were seen as agitation, mental deterioration and indolence. The latter term was an unusual one to use but it referred to an enforced indolence, not one of personal choice, and this led to boredom and apathy as well as withdrawal. The social complications centered around losses; of friendship, roles, family and interaction. This, in turn, led to humiliation, distrust, mental deterioration, social isolation, cognitive deprivation and abnormal social behaviour. **Figure 1** on page 16 depicts the tree that McIver used as a metaphor for custodial care.[14]

As she reviewed the film clips, McIver was encouraged by the transformation in the *residents* (no longer called patients) after only a few months of what she was calling Restorative Care. She dreamed of a healthy tree in which all the roots were well nourished by a variety of holistic care approaches. If this could be attained, the branches and leaves of the tree would blossom leading to independence and the attainment of a strong social, personal, and spiritual identity for the person (see **Figure 2** on page 17).[15] In this healthy tree there were many programmes in place. Using McIver's detailed vision of the tree we were able to compile **Table 1** on page 18 which shows how the programmes of care could lead to the fruits and more desirable overall outcomes for the residents. These programmes are elaborated on in chapter 3.

---

[14]   Wing, D. (2003). Adapted from McIver, V., Patrick, G., & Dolny, J. (1972, June). Custodial Care Tree. Unpublished drawing. Victoria, BC

[15]   Wing, D. (2003). Adapted from McIver, V., Patrick, G., & Dolny, J. (1972, June). Restorative Care Tree. Unpublished drawing. Victoria, BC.

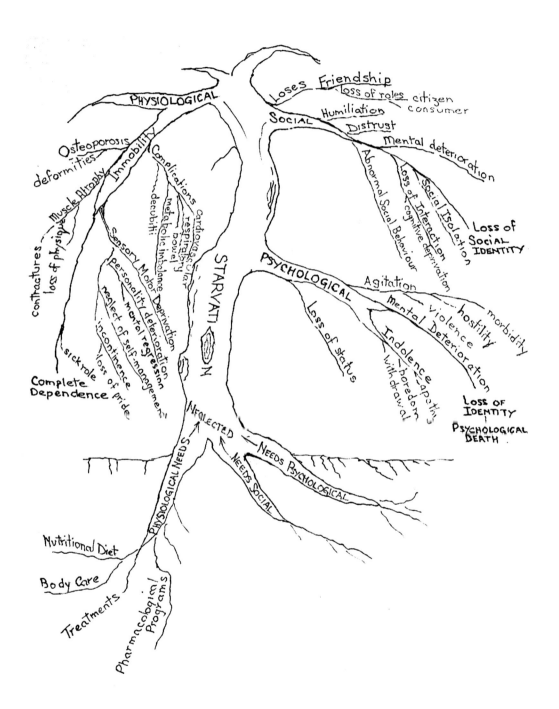

Figure 1 Custodial Care

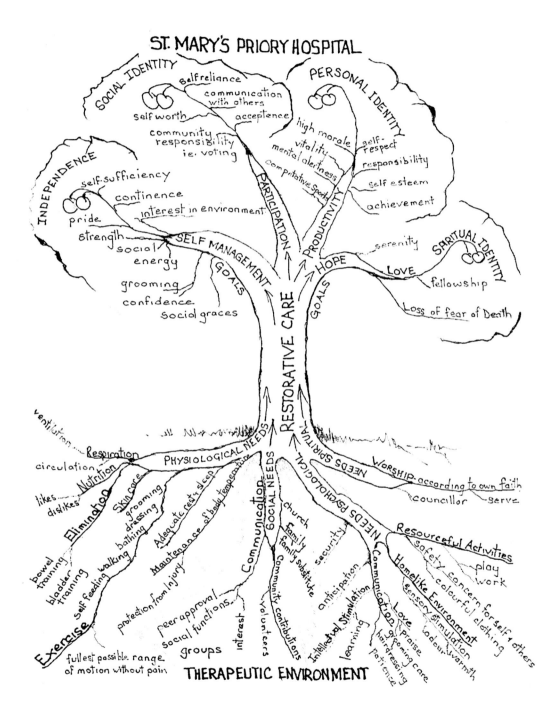

Figure 2 Restorative Care

Table I
Restorative Care Programme as Visualized in the Tree[16]

ROOTS OF THE TREE (Needs)	NUTRIENTS (programmes of care)	LIMBS AND BRANCHES (Intermediate Outcomes)	FRUITS OF THE TREE (End States)
PHYSIOLOGICAL NEEDS e.g Respiration, nutrition, mobility, safety etc.	STRENGTHENING THE BODY e.g Breathing exercises, bowel & bladder training, skin care programme, exercise acitivities in grooming, dressing, bathing, walking, self-feeding	SELF MANAGEMENT Interest in the environment Social graces Energy Strength Continence Confidence in grooming Pride Self sufficiency	INDEPENDENCE
PSYCHOLOGICAL NEEDS e.g. self esteem, ego strength, self respect	STRENGTHENING THE EGO e.g. fostering Communication opportunities, offering freedom of choice, resourceful activities (play, work, fostering concern for others) CREATING COMMUNITY e.g. bus for outings, volunteers, use of service clubs, family nights	PRODUCTIVITY Achievement Self-esteem Responsibility Self respect Competitive sport Mental alertness Vitality High morale	SENSE OF PERSONAL IDENTITY
SOCIAL NEEDS e.g. sense of belonging,	HUMANIZING THE LIVING SPACE e.g. interest groups leading to Peer group approval and social functioning , home-like environment CREATING COMMUNITY	PARTICIPATION Acceptance Communication with others Community responsibilities Feelings of self-worth Self reliance	SENSE OF SOCIAL IDENTITY
SPIRITUAL NEEDS	ALL THE ABOVE PROGRAMMES *and* Worship opportunities, Memorial services	HOPE Love Fellowship Loss of fear of death Serenity	SENSE OF SPIRITUAL IDENTITY

[16]   Mantle, J. (2003). Analysis of the Tree Drawing. Victoria, BC.

McIver Remembers the Development of the Tree Metaphor.

One day I saw a picture of a beautiful green tree, but the roots were exposed. This gave me an inspiration – I transposed this thought to human needs. The roots of the tree represented the basic needs of the older person-physiological, psychological and spiritual. The trunk was the channel through which sustenance from the roots nourished the branches and leaves. Independence and identity (social, personal and spiritual) were the fruits. If the roots were inadequately fed, the tree would not receive the necessary nutrients and would not flourish. When I reviewed the earlier film clips what I saw was that the individual who had been receiving custodial care was like a starving tree that was misshapen, distorted by losses caused by starvation and at risk of dying. I reasoned that this came about because there was only minimal attention being given to the life-sustaining roots. This neglect leads to the starvation of trunk and limbs resulting in a multiplicity of life-draining problems. Only some of the basic physiological needs were receiving any attention at all. Through providing a nutritious diet, giving body care, and by implementing medical treatments and pharmacological management, nourishment of only the most basic kind was provided. Thus I drew this picture of deprivation in the tree (Figure 1). This became the blue print upon which care could be developed.

(McIver, V. 2001. Personal Interview)

The tree became the medium through which McIver could teach Restorative Care. For the first "People Tree" workshop a portable symbolic tree was created. Streamers flowing down from a tree displayed the roots. Flowers and colorful leaves marked the fruits on the tree. The physiological roots led to a tray with a tea service, simple exercise equipment, canes and crutches and grooming items. The roots of social and spiritual needs led to a small church. Where an object could not be depicted a picture was placed on a card to denote the intent. For example, family was shown in a picture with grandparents, children and adults. In showing the psychological needs, the motivating forces were printed on cards. The model became the focus of staff inservice education as well as being used in workshops and orienting professional visitors to the concepts. The tree model also informed the general public when it was featured in a front window at Eaton's Department Store.

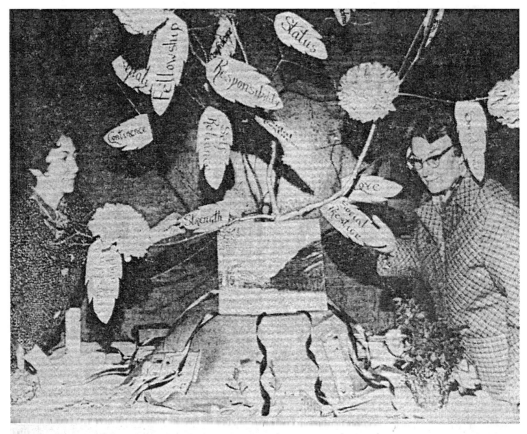

People Tree Workshop Popular

Workshop for volunteers interested in elderly persons drew 225 participants at day-long training event in First United Church this week. Standing by People Tree, which gave workshop its name, are, left, Mrs. Leona Aitken, who worked as guide, and Gertrude Patmore, registrar.—(Ellis Shipman)

<u>Daily Colonist</u>, April, 1973, Victoria, B.C.

PHILOSOPHY OF THE PRIORY RESTORATIVE CARE MODEL

McIver had a keen sense of what needed to be done and one could say that, at first, she had an intuitive philosophy. However when one of the nurses that worked at the Priory returned from a conference, she advised that there was a need for a written statement about the philosophy. McIver set about this task and asked the staff to help by providing ideas. When nothing was forthcoming, McIver and Harrison (the administrator) sat down over a cup of tea and the ideas flowed.

The philosophy they wrote had three main elements as shown below.[17]

We believe in the dignity and worth of all human beings.

In order to make this a viable fact within a total community, all staff - with the resident and his family - develop a restorative program. Together, all are given the opportunity to reach and attain their maximum potential in the pursuit of growth and development.

With the freedom of expression, encouragement and a positive expectation, all strive toward a continuum of care, which encompasses prevention and maintains, improves or restores bio-psycho-social health.

For McIver a philosophy was acted out through a combination of clinical and administrative behaviors. In an unpublished paper she wrote:

> As with any enterprise, one establishes a strong foundation upon which to build an effective organization. The foundation stone is a central philosophy expressing the collective values of the professional and non-professional membership. Then you establish an effective structure to support this philosophy. Attempting to make this a reality is a very exciting experience and privilege.[18]

Williamson, a British nurse on a study tour in Canada in 1976-78, observed that this model of care was not focused on facilities, manpower or money but rather on quality of care and service provided. In his report of his visits he observed "there was within this setting an abstract, intangible factor that the Priory Hospital seems to embrace and impart to both staff and residents who worked or lived within this environment."[19] The authors suggest that what he was observing and experiencing was the powerful effects of a philosophy being lived out in the daily actions of all the staff and people who entered the facility.

---

[17] Williamson, F. (1978). <u>A Psychosocial Model of Health Care: The Priory Concept - a Baseline Approach: An Environment for Long-Term Care: A Canadian Nursing Study Review</u>. Unpublished monograph prepared as a result of a Florence Nightingale Scholarship. England. 2.

[18] McIver, V. (1977, July), <u>Humanizing the workplace</u>. Unpublished paper. Victoria, BC.

[19] Williamson, F. (1978). ix.

chapter 3

Restorative Care Practice

In this chapter we will discuss the guiding ideas underlying Restorative Care and follow this with a description of the clinical approaches used in Restorative Care practice. We identify the fundamental elements that served to orient the staff in their new practice. We highlight the approaches developed for the special situations of dementia and dying in the elderly and we conclude with a discussion of the particular strategies used to implement the programmes. It was these components that made Restorative Care at the Priory significantly different from the usual care practices offered in other like facilities of that time.

GUIDING IDEAS IN RESTORATIVE CARE

In Restorative Care five critical overall strategies were linked together to direct the care programmes.

- The whole person rather than just their disability became the focus of attention.
- The total environment, including staff behaviors, was re-designed to convey positive expectations of wellness and the maximum use of remaining abilities.[20] The Priory became a community within itself and a participating member of the larger community outside.
- The institution was de-institutionalized through humanizing the hospital environment.
- The activities of daily living were normalized, particularly through environmental changes and strengthening the body.
- An interdependency model of care was adopted where the residents were supported by staff to carry out their own activities of daily living, thus strengthening their ego.[21]

---

[20]   Williamson, F. (1978). <u>A Psychosocial Model of Health Care: The Priory Concept - a Baseline Approach: An Environment for Long-Term Care: A Canadian Nursing Study Review</u>. Unpublished monograph prepared as a result of a Florence Nightingale Scholarship. England. x.

[21]   Williamson, F. (1978). 46.

In this model, particular clinical and management acts, either alone or in combination, were seen to achieve multiple goals. The reverse was also true and to achieve any particular goal you needed multiple interventions. Later in this chapter we have used summary charts to demonstrate some of the strategies used by the staff. The reader will note the overlap of actions in the charts revealing how a particular action can meet several goals.

The blending of strategies to meet a goal is exemplified by the way in which the eating routine was normalized. McIver had observed that many of the residents were not able to feed themselves and had regressed to eating pureed food. She recalls:

> A resident's apathy toward feeding himself is frequently seen and follows a pattern. This indifference is more pronounced where the resident eats in his own bed, off a tray without social interaction. The resident begins to toy with the food, eating less and less, when this persists, the nurse gives help in order to get sufficient caloric intake. This of course does not improve the situation; the resident hasn't the appetite, is too weak, and forgets how to feed herself. It becomes a downward spiral because the feeding is so time consuming, [and] the nurse resorts to pureed food as it goes down more easily.[22]

The road back to self-feeding was slow, but setting up an enabling environment that was more normal was the goal. For the residents, this included getting up out of bed, being appropriately dressed and joining in mealtime conversations with others around a familiar dining room setting. The creation of a family style dining room (communal) where residents no longer had to eat from a tray while in bed or at the bedside was a critical environmental change. Some brief pre-mealtime entertainment was started. The tables were attractively set and mealtime was treated as a special time for residents. The food was not served on institutional-like trays. It was plated from heated bulk food containers directly in front of the residents with the kitchen staff dressed as Chefs and having direct contact and conversation with the residents as to likes and dislikes. Eventually those residents who were capable were given food in bowls and platters for self-serving. These residents served themselves and helped other residents who needed assistance to fill their plates. The physical environmental changes helped to maintain good eating habits that strengthened the body as well as providing opportunity for normal socialization. The reaching for and passing of food provided exercise as well as opportunities for personal decision-making about what to eat and identifying who needed help. By helping others, residents were able to meet their own psychosocial needs for belong-

---

[22] McIver, V. (1969, April). Communal dining : Idea exchange. <u>Canadian Nurse Journal</u>, 65(4). 45.

ing and doing meaningful work. There was also the provision of a kitchenette for residents and family's use.[23] This provided the residents and/or families with a way of participating in meaningful familiar social activities, in a homelike setting. It provided an outlet for the need to perform domestic duties, as well as care giving through preparation of tea and baked goodies when residents and /or family members were capable to do so. Those that were able would also wash their own dishes and tidy up.

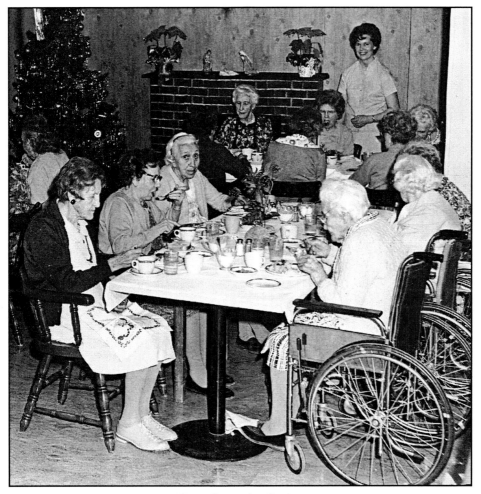

Family style dining

---

[23]   McIver V. (1972, December). For a more human approach to long-term patient care. Hospital Administration in Canada, 55-57.

Four fundamental elements formed the basis of Restorative Care practice. Activities centered on *strengthening the body* became the first order of business so that the older people had enough energy and physical ability to move forward toward the highest level of wellness that they could achieve. The focus *on strengthening the ego, humanizing the living space,* and *creating the Priory as a community,* nourished the psychological, social, and spiritual roots of the person. The special situations of *dementia* and *dying* were addressed by particular programming. Finally these areas were sustained by *changes in the method of practice.* **Figure 3** illustrates Restorative Care and its fundamental elements. The elements have been transplanted on to the tree used by McIver in the metaphor described earlier and are elaborated on below.

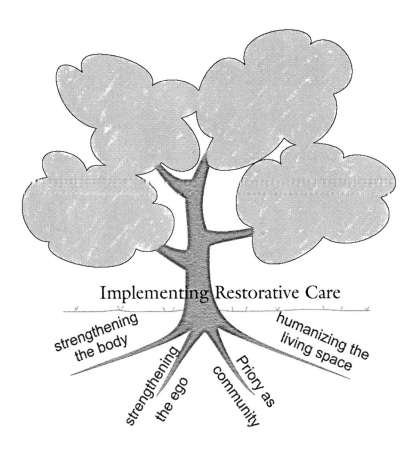

Figure 3. *Fundamental elements of restorative care*

AREAS OF FOCUS IN RESTORATIVE CARE

1. Strengthening the Body

Mobility became the key to unlocking the doors of the world from which the older people had been removed by custodial care. Gaining muscle strength and using substitutive devices for weakness was the key to that mobility. With an increased budget, wheelchairs were provided and residents were enabled to participate in many functions. The wheelchair was used only for mobility and when the residents were up, they were seated in ordinary chairs or participating in a walking programme. Walkers and canes were issued for those who could benefit from them. Initially the residents were very weak and before the staff could remove restraints completely, seatbelt-like restraints were used for wheelchairs to assist in supporting them in an upright position.

An activity coordinator was hired to establish an activity programme. Exercises to strengthen muscles and limber joints were started. From McIver's point of view exercises should be an enjoyable experience and performed within a social milieu, perhaps accompanied by music. Initially they were begun in bed and then followed later by the use of parallel handrails for relearning to walk. A single exercise might accomplish several purposes. She saw that tossing a ball back and forth could both strengthen muscles and help to co-ordinate movements. Being able to coordinate one's movements was necessary to manipulate food to the mouth and resume a more normal eating pattern. Purposeful activities such as ringing out the washcloth, making cookies and sewing were useful in fostering finger dexterity and providing hand exercises.[24]

Rather than using expensive equipment, exercises were built into all activities throughout the day.[25] All nursing staff became involved in walking and range-of-motion exercises. The use of catheters was reduced by planning routine toileting, and those residents who could walk with an assistant were expected to walk to the toilets.[26] This approach also had a positive effect on the budget by reducing linen costs by $28,000 per year per 100 residents. Tossing a ball or beanbags into a basket would limber the joints and also avoid boredom. The residents participated in arts and crafts to assist the ladies auxiliary in preparation for a bazaar and a luau further exercising their limbs and joints.

---

[24] McIver, V. (1974, September 6). Reactivation to Self-Feeding. Speech given at the Priory Hospital, Victoria, BC. 3.

[25] McIver, V. (1973, February). A New Environment for Extended Care. Proceedings of the Seminar on Extended Care, British Columbia Hospitals' Association. Richmond, BC. 39.

[26] McIver, V. (1971, July). Reap Your Own Harvest. Unpublished paper.

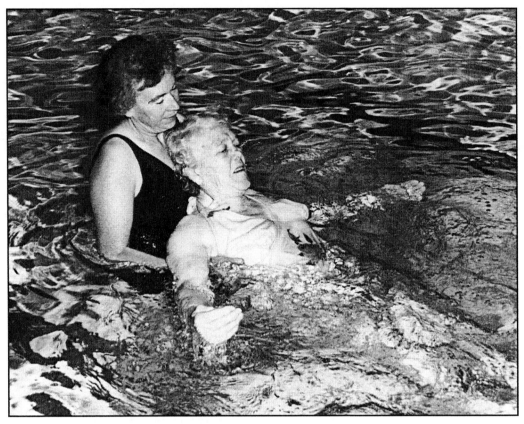

Resident enjoying a swim at the local recreation centre.

SAMPLE ACTIVITIES FOR STRENGTHENING THE BODY

- Removed catheters
- Began toileting programme
- Resident walked to exercises
- Self-feeding
- Wheelchairs for mobility and participation in all activities
- Exercises incorporated into daily living activities
- New beds replaced cots and could be rolled up
- Hoyer lifts
- Through family style dining residents passed food and got exercise at the same time
- Games and crafts

2. Strengthening the Ego

Psychological rehabilitation was seen to add quality of life to the resident's remaining years.[27] Efforts were made to foster relationships of caring. Staff, families, visitors and volunteers of all ages and sexes as well as pets helped to provide the needed friendship and enhance the residents' sense of dignity, worth, self-esteem, ego integrity and identity.[28] McIver used the term "active friendliness" to show the resident that the staff really cared and were willing to give support, encouragement and friendship. Staff was advised to liberally use ego enhancers such as praise, understanding, encouragement, sincere flattery, and the granting of wishes and desires.[29]

Establishing these relationships was a new challenge for the staff because the idea of moving into friendships with their residents was a complete break with the hospital tradition of maintaining remote professional relationships. It was McIver's view that staff attitudes and behavior directly affected how the residents felt about themselves. She saw that "ego-building experiences had to be deliberately planned but allowed to happen in a spontaneity of fellowship".[30] All staff were educated to convey positive expectations toward maximum use of the residents' remaining abilities.

In order to foster an individual's desire and ability to participate in their care and in their world, a variety of techniques were introduced. Using a board with day, date, weather and holidays fostered a *Reality Orientation*. Clocks with large numbers were hung in strategic places. Residents were called by name in all groups. *Remotivation* therapy focused on evoking healthy aspects of the personality was instituted. *Sensory Stimulation* with a special emphasis on touch was incorporated into everyday living, as were the other modalities.

Reminiscing was combined with *oral histories* in a very creative way. Funding was obtained to write a book based on the oral histories of the residents. It was printed and dedicated to all those who had made the Priory Hospital a reality.[31] The women who contributed to the book had experienced varying hardships including child labor in the coal mines in Wales, bombing in two world wars, pioneer life on the prairies, the great depression and drought on the prairies. They told stories about the new Ford and the introduction of telephones and

---

[27] McIver, V. (1976, November). With Dignity and Respect. Notes of a speech given at the University Of Victoria, Victoria, BC.

[28] Saunders, P. (1976). Lesson 12, Section IV: Specific Implementation of Concepts. Programme Manual. Unpublished. 19.

[29] St Mary's Priory Hospital. (1970, June). Job Description – Care Coordinator.

[30] McIver, V. (1974, September 6). Reactivation to Self-Feeding. Speech presented at The Priory Hospital, Victoria, BC. 2.

[31] Bambiger, B & Milord, J. (Eds). (1975). Gifts of Aging: An Anthology of the Human Journey. Unpublished.

THE LEADER-POST, REGINA, SASK. JUNE 29, 1977

Patient's emotional needs stressed

By RUTH WARICK
Of Staff Reporter

The film shows an elderly woman hauling out Hallowe'en treats to youngsters dressed as witches, cats, cowboys and other make-believe characters.

There is nothing extraordinary about that, except the scene takes place in a hospital and at one time the patient would have had a difficult, if not impossible, time being mobile. She is an example of patients participating in an extended-care program for the elderly in St. Mary's Priory Hospital in Victoria.

The film, shown to the 50 nurses attending a two-day workshop sponsored by the Saskatchewan Registered Nurses' Association in the Regina Inn last week, was presented by Mrs. Vera McIver, director of services at St. Mary's Priory Hospital. The workshop was held Tuesday.

In an interview, Mrs. McIver said a hospital is an environment for people who must remain in for long periods of time. "The institu-

tion is built, not to accommodate the patient, but for the patient to accommodate himself to it.

"The hospital is no place for elderly people. It's for people who stay only five days, then leave. It is a terrible tragedy what we do to them (older people)."

She said patients are given a good diet, good body care and pills and it is generally thought they are getting good care. But their social, psychological and spiritual needs are forgotten.

The situation is more acute for long-term patients because they are removed from their normal social contacts in society. They need to have a new identity and feel loved and wanted. They need new contacts, Mrs. McIver said.

"Too often patients are put in a bed and must play the sick role. They are made to be dependent on the hospital, eventually are fed by a spoon and use a bedpan. They begin to deteriorate both mentally and physically."

Mrs. McIver said nurses and doctors are trained, not to give bedside comfort, but to be highly technical and work-orientated.

"The approach is happy when she can approach the patient with her props, a hypo to give or a blood pressure to take. She never has time to hold a hand or give an ear."

But there is hope.

Mrs. McIver said there is a trend to extended-care homes, where attempts are being made to meet the patient's emotional as well as physical needs. St. Mary's Priory Hospital was the leader in this relatively new development, she said.

Five years ago, Mrs. McIver planned to retire to Victoria with her husband. Born in Avonlea, she graduated from Regina Grey Nuns Hospital in 1941 and worked off and on as a nurse until the early 1960s. Her plans for retirement were cut short when her sister asked her to pull up the standards of St. Mary's

Priory, to meet government regulations. The hospital had just come under government control.

"I really thought I was descending, to go to St. Mary's, but I did it—please my sister."

Mrs. McIver became a key figure in developing an extended service which meets the patient's emotional, as well as physical needs. There are now 85 extended-care patients in 85. Last year the hospital received accreditation under the Canadian Council on Hospital Accreditation which recommended it be used as an educational source example to other units.

Activities in the unit are varied, but the two basics are that patients are encouraged to eat with each other in a dining room and in bedrooms. They sing songs, cook, sew on one of six buttons, engage in seal activities, go to beauty parlors, wear "pretty clothes," go outside for tea and into the community. Around Christmas time they go out to vote, Mrs. McIver said.

Volunteers are used heavily, providing patients with much needed outside contact, she added.

Mrs. McIver said it does not take any more money to provide love and attention. The use of volunteers can do much, too. For example, the hospital uses an average of 13 pounds of linen per patient per day—because patients are able to use the washroom—compared to 31 pounds used in most hospitals.

"This is a saving of $28,000 a year per 100 patients, she said.

Mrs. McIver said it doesn't take any more time for a nurse to have a pleasant conversation with a patient while waiting her turn at it than to keep a stony silence.

She said it may be easier to feed the patient and bring the bedpan around, but in the end the dependent patient will require more care than a self-sufficient one.

Mrs. McIver feels some of the radical changes necessary to improve care for the old must come within the educational system of nurses and doctors. She believes more emphasis must be placed on restorative and rehabilitative training, and more social services classes must be offered.

She also feels the whole area of long-term patient care and uplifting so hospitals and nurses will not look upon it as the least important aspect of medical care.

Often, well-trained nurses will not go into the area because it has low prestige.

In addition, she feels hospital structures should be broken away from home for patients. She favors separation of extended-care services because it allows nurses to be trained to care for these patients will usually not be able to adapt to a different attitude needed to treat extended-care patients.

Mrs. McIver also favors more government support so that nursing homes can maintain a consistent, high standard. While they care for a patient's social needs, attention to the emotional well-being is lacking in most nursing

A NURSE'S SMILE. Mrs. Vera McIver, director of services at St. Mary's Althouse Hospital in Victoria, smiles as she shows some of the patients in the extended-care program. Although they average 85 years of age, the patients actively engage in social and recreational activities under a special program developed at the hospital. The film was one of the features of the Saskatchewan Registered Nurses Association in the Regina Inn last week. Mrs. McIver is a graduate of Regina Grey Nuns Hospital and worked as a nurse in the early 1940s and became a member...

THE PROVINCE, Saturday, December 11, 1971 ★★★41

Woman's Province

Mind care comes first

Unlike the traditional rest-homes for the aged, St. Mary's Priory in Victoria is a place old people go to live, not wait for death. In this third of a three part series, KAY ALSOP explains why.

VICTORIA: A cluster of unpretentious wooden buildings here houses Canada's outstanding extended care facility.

St. Mary's Priory Hospital, recently awarded full accreditation by the Canadian Council, has been credited by consultant Nicole Du Mouchel, R.N., M.N., with being the equal of New York's Loeb Centre, formerly considered the most progressive nursing centre on the continent.

Dr. Floris King, co-ordinator of graduate programs, and associate professor of U.B.C.'s School of Nursing, praises the Priory for "the very special way it attacks the problems associated with extended care."

"You don't need a palace," says Vera McIver, director of the hospital's services. "Desire is all that it takes to make an improvement."

Dr. King goes further, crediting Mrs. McIver's keenness, her vitality and initiative, and her courage to act, for much of the success of the Priory Method of remotivation.

There was, for instance, the color-coding of doors. No

numbers. Instead, the individual doors along the corridors are painted bright yellows, or oranges, or pinks, or blues, or turquoises or greens, and little old ladies look for their own color, and don't have to ask a nurse to help them locate themselves, which is good for their independence.

The whole hospital is as bright and gay as a flower garden — "we went all out for color to make everybody feel happy," says Mrs. McIver. "With old people we have to stimulate all the senses.

"A drab, sterile environment encourages the sick role and social isolation. It is not only untherapeutic, it is antitherapeutic. Therefore, to enhance the visual surroundings, every effort should be made to introduce change, warmth and color. This, then, becomes a source of stimulation and motivation because it triggers the brain thought mechanism and promotes involvement rather than withdrawal."

A beautiful environment benefits in a great many ways, according to experts like Louis E. Gelwicks, research associate of the Gerontology Center, University of

Southern California, who recommends the carpeting of private rooms in extended care hospitals as an aid against incontinence, for example.

He emphasizes the use of space, deplores the abuse of multi-purpose rooms, as ideas Mrs. McIver who claims that it's confusing to elderly residents to be put in dual purpose environments. She cites examples — toilets and commodes in a place other than a bathroom (which lack of space makes necessary at the Priory unfortunately), or a makeshift chapel set up and knocked down in the corner of a gym.

Both Mrs. McIver and Lillian McLean, R.N., hospital services director of Vancouver's Louis Brier Home, have decided opinions on the construction of extended care units.

For one thing, says Mrs. McLean, they should be freestanding, not part of an acute care establishment, because the philosophy from the one spills over onto the other. Doctors and nurses who are "O.R."-orientated find it difficult to think in terms of remotivation for the elderly, tend to administer pills instead of interest of a more social nature.

"If people would only think of extended care as an extension of the home, not the hospital, part of our problem would be solved," she says.

Both Mrs. McLean and Mrs. McIver stress the need for architects and planners of extended care units to consult nurses as to the practicability of their designs.

with the facilities all the time," they say. "Strange as it may seem, hospitals and homes for the aged have actually been built without radiators in the bathrooms, or ramps in the doorways for wheelchairs. It's the little things which make all the difference.

"If you take the advice of nurses in the beginning you save on the cost of bedside care later, because experienced nurses know immediately how to save lives," says Mrs. McLean. It makes a great difference — a building poorly laid out could require 3.5 nursing hours per patient per day in order to give proper care, whereas the government recommends (as a guide line) 2.5 nursing hours per patient a day. The slack, say the ladies, is taken up by denying the patient.

Mrs. McIver tells about one extended care home where the residents slumped dispiritedly in chairs, or simply stayed in bed. The windowsills were so high they couldn't see out, she says. No chance to watch a bird sitting through the trees. No way to laugh at children playing in the park. Not even an opportunity to keep track of visitors coming and going.

And that's another very important point, says Mrs. McLean. Visitors are so essential to older people that all extended care homes should have plenty of accessible, and preferably free, parking.

But even inadequate facilities can be overcome if the nurses understand the impor-

"It takes longer to re-educate the staff sometimes than to remotivate patients," says George Harrison, administrator of St. Mary's Priory Hospital. He often has to remind new nurses that "that patient you just went roaring past wanted to talk to you."

"Nurses are often afraid of a person-to-person involvement," says Vera McIver. "They're more confident of their own role if they're dealing with a sick person — they're trained to be so acute-minded it's hard for them to change.

shows more concern that the patient's bed is properly made and the castors kicked into place than she does about her patient's sense of individual worth," says Mrs. McIver. "She's got to become aware that, without the right attitude on her part, she can break a patient's heart, destroy her identity, vegetate her life.

"At St. Mary's Priory Hospital we shower our ladies with love. They are dear to us and we let them know it. They have responded to this spirit of affection with a new awakening."

more people who need long term care", concludes Dr. Floris King. Which means that the need for greater understanding of the requirements of extended care is becoming imperative, in her estimation.

"Let's get a study going", she urges. "That might help to trigger things right across Canada. Goodness knows, we've got a shining example of what extended care COULD be right here in British Columbia."

Vera McIver smiles her quiet smile.

Mrs. Helen McCloy and nurse Jean Brailsford keep up to date.

radios. They had used oxen in the fields and now saw men on the moon. Everyone who contributed (residents, families and staff) felt they had contributed to a worthwhile project – an ego-enhancing experience for all concerned.

McIver looked at ways of removing barriers to normal functioning by renovating toilets and bathing rooms for easy access and by increasing the numbers of toilets and commodes. When residents were no longer incontinent and had leisurely and soothing bathing experiences their physical functions as well as self-esteem improved.

SAMPLE ACTIVITIES FOR STRENGTHENING THE EGO

• Creating caring relationships with staff, families, visitors, volunteers – Active friendliness	• Reality Orientation
	• Remotivation therapy
	• Sensory Stimulation with emphasis on touch
• Welcoming of pets to the facility	
• Staff education to convey positive expectations of resident's remaining abilities	• Reminiscing
	• Removing barriers to normal functioning
• Generous use of ego enhancers e.g. praise, understanding, encouragement	e.g. renovating baths and toilets

3. Humanizing the Living Space

McIver was persuaded that the environment, a term she used in the broadest sense, had a powerful effect on human behavior - residents, families, and staff. She wrote:

> This acute care model with its impersonal, mechanical and dehumanizing care [is] seen to create an anti therapeutic environment for extended care people. Little wonder then that our professional institutional environment can destroy human dignity and replace it with vegetation in a person who is deprived of adequate emotional and social care.[32]

---

[32]   McIver, V. (1973, February). A New Environment for Extended Care. Proceedings of the Seminar on Extended Care. British Columbia Hospitals' Association. Richmond, BC. 40.

Humanizing the living space and making it home-like was the medium for moving away from the acute care model. McIver believed that the environment of institutional long-term care settings should recognize individuals as feeling, intelligent and capable human beings.[33] Meaningful work/play, cultural enrichment and opportunity for expression of spiritual and altruistic values were seen to be essential to all persons in this environment.[34]

A Story of Meaningful Work Achieving Multiple Goals[35]

In early spring a baby lamb was brought in to be cuddled and fed from the bottle. The lamb visited on numerous occasions, so it had to have a name. A "Name the Lamb" contest was held and the name chosen was "Gladys." When Gladys became an adult and shearing time came around, it was done at the Priory. Gladys was bathed and a week later she was shorn with the wool donated to the ladies. What would they do with the wool? It was decided to make a quilt. They had to tease the wool in preparation for the quilt. This work lasted three months and was truly built-in exercise. They purchased the material and since they had their own treadle sewing machine, they exercised once more while sewing the pockets that would hold the wool. Once filled, the quilt was sewn together. It was decided to raffle the quilt. Tickets were made and sold. They realized close to $400. Our staff was always very generous in enterprises that raised money for a cause. Discussions now followed about what to do with the money. They decided to buy a china cabinet for the activity room.

A delegation was taken to a furniture store and the choice was made for a nice cabinet with a beautiful hutch. Unfortunately it was over $800. One of the ladies asked to see the manager and negotiated the price they could afford along with free delivery. It was decided to hold a tea with the admission price to be a china teacup and saucer to display in the cabinet. The staff helped the residents prepare the tea and the teacakes and sandwiches. On the day of the party a resident who had been severely withdrawn and had not participated up to this time, took a sandwich when it was passed and ate it. The environment took her back to another time when she knew what was expected of her. All this was the offshoot of a visiting lamb named Gladys.

---

[33] Warick, R. (1972, June). Patient's emotional needs stressed. Leader Post. Regina, Sask. 11.
[34] McIver, V. (1973, February). 40.
[35] McIver, V. (1999). Unpublished manuscript. 71.

Since the word 'patient' denoted an illness, it was decided to use the word 'resident' as more reflective of the new image. In addition, nursing staff began calling each other by their first names and residents who preferred this familiarity were also called by their first names. This action tended to produce a sense of camaraderie among everyone in the home-like setting. [36]

McIver worked with the staff in the adoption of home-like wearing apparel. Staff stopped wearing white, clinical looking uniforms, and wore casual dress. Staff in uniforms conveyed an institutional milieu and levels of status, and therefore civilian clothes for all was deemed to be more appropriate as it overcame the professional aura, which tends to inhibit communication.[37] The more casual attire affected the social and psychological milieu and reduced the institutional and dependent nature of social interaction. The kitchen staff wore aprons and chef hats as they do in hotel services.

Visiting hours were unrestricted allowing people to come and go freely. The coffeepot was always on, free of charge, to all family and volunteers. With their newfound abilities allowing them to join in activities, residents were able to meet their needs for socialization and human contact. This allowed them to play their former roles as much as possible and spouses, children, grandchildren and friends were welcomed to the Priory Hospital.

The physical interior structures and furnishings of the facility underwent changes. Nursing workstations became more like offices where staff could chart or use the telephone to call the physician. McIver had learned from her reading that humans deteriorate when they lack sufficient sensory stimulation and that "color can introduce sensory stimulation, break up monotony, and establish an interesting change of pace."[38] Thus renovations included the use of bright cheerful colors in the painting of walls and decorating of rooms, a change from the commonly used institutional green. Resident bedrooms were decorated with colorful bed throws, afghans, pillows and curtains. Pegboards and shelves at each bedside were helpful for tacking up personal cards and pictures. Full spectrum lighting replaced fluorescent lights because she had read about the positive changes in reproduction habits of confined animals under these conditions.

Outdoor wheelchair-accessible leisure spaces were established for residents. These were used for activities such as gardening, recreational activities, and picnics. They provided both stimulation and meaningful familiar experiences for the residents and their families and the sun was a great therapeutic resource.

[36] McIver, V. (1973, February). A New Environment for Extended Care. Proceedings of the Seminar on Extended Care. British Columbia Hospitals' Association. Richmond, BC. 40.

[37] Dunsmuir, A. (1973, April). Seniors gain fuller lives when wards lose starch, The Colonist. Victoria, BC.

[38] Birren, T. (1970). Color for Interiors - Historical and Modern. New York: Whitney Publications Inc. 131.

Daily Colonist, Victoria, B.

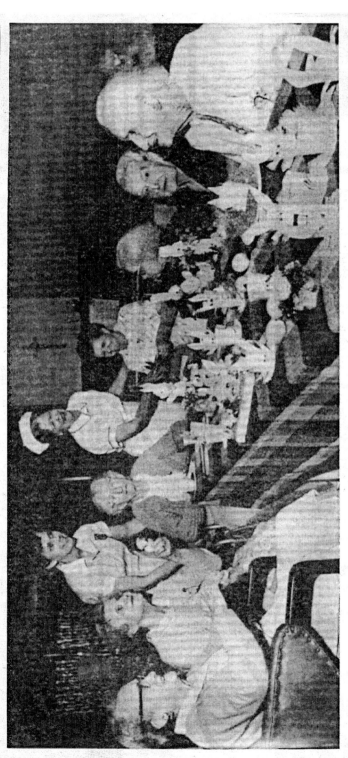

Remotivation Key Word in B.C. Scheme

Patients Find New Goals

BY DON GAIN

A heartwarming story came out of St. Mary's Priory at Colwood this week.

It told of the miracle of spring and Easter in the

care hospitals, mostly older people, who require specialized nursing care.

"We are trying to provide a greater breadth of activities for them to ensure that they

Mrs. McIver listed some of the programmed activities which have had beneficial effects on the patients' welfare — speech therapy, handicrafts, singing.

atmosphere of support for these people. It had helped them to regain their independence."

The current project is one with an Easter flavor. A

so doing, might reawaken spring in their own hearts."

"We've all got a vested interest in old age," Mr. Giles said. "We're all heading in that direction."

Purposeful People

Mrs. Joan Dolny, occupational therapist, and Nurse Ethehl Drewery inspect Easter novelties made by, from left, Mrs. Marguerite LaTullippe, Mrs. Bertha Stradiotto, Mrs. Emma Quick, Miss Phyllis Kerr, Mrs. Victoria Taylor, Mrs. Hannah Cullington and Mrs. Clara Livingston.—(Robin Clarke)

The Province, December 10, 1971

Woman's Province

LEARNING TO ENJOY LIVING AGAIN BASIS OF PRIORY METHODS

The therapy of doing

VICTORIA: Vera McIver, director of hospital services at St. Mary's Priory Hospital, is smiling as she leads the way down the colorful corridors of this 95 bed extended care haven for elderly ladies.

"You'd be surprised how little our program costs, because we just make use of everyday living experiences," she says.

Simple therapy like letting the ladies bake and decorate birthday cakes for each other, or encouraging them to plan menus, cook the food and set the table for luncheon parties, gears up excitement, enhances egos when the results are openly appreciated and applauded by the staff and fellow residents.

"We encourage them to look after their own clothes," says Mrs. McIver, "so they sew their own buttons on, if at all possible, and they use the old treadle sewing machine to do mending, and run up gift items. Again, it's a familiar skill, it's creative, gives them a feeling of usefulness — but best of all, it's an excellent way for them to exercise their legs and arms."

Other simple exercises may include w a t e r i n g plants, changing the dates in the calendar — simple, everyday things which require a little effort, yield a sense of accomplishment and purpose.

When deterioration of the body and mind in the aged is due to neglect it can be reversed, as proved by the Priory Method. But before a remotivation program can be initiated, the staff must recognize and be convinced of the need for rehabilitative care, instead of the traditional acute hospital care. This is all-important, because if the emphasis is placed on the sick role and the patient is given only custodial care, she will experience a loss of identity and with it, deterioration.

"People play the roles assigned to them," says Vera McIver.

When its remotivation program was initiated four years ago, the Priory listed 95 women on its resident list. Most were over the age of 85. Most were seriously impaired.

The first step was to get them mobile, through individually planned exercises, so they could have their meals in the communal dining room instead of in bed, so they could go to the bathroom instead of using a bedpan, two factors contributing to their personal sickroom image.

At first only five of the residents had their meals in the dining room. W i t h i n six months the situation had completely reversed, and there were only five still having their meals on a tray in their beds. The same kind of Great Expectations held true in the matter of toilet training.

"It's so easy to just take

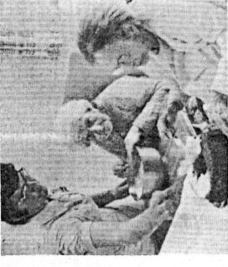

Nurse Sally Surette, Mrs. Millicent Sanders and Mrs. Dorothy Carnie . . . getting ready for a party.

to a bed. At the Priory we do consistent toileting. It takes patience and time, but it is worth it in more ways than one.

"Some extended care units use 12 pounds of linen per patient, per day. At the Priory, we average 4.5 pounds, which means a financial saving in laundry of something like $28,000 a year."

Once they're not soiling their clothes, the ladies can be encouraged to wear pretty dresses and think about personal grooming, and that involves therapy of two kinds, active and mental.

There's the physical exercise involved in dressing themselves, in going to the

perms, comb-outs and make-up. And there's the exhilaration and pride of self which comes out of a "pretty lady" image instead of a colorless, invalid reflection in the mirror.

The very act of eating is used in the remotivation program at the Priory, and sparks a chain reaction of improvement in the individual residents.

"It's much easier for a nurse to feed older people osterited food at their bedside," says Mrs. McIver. "But if they can be encouraged to eat with a spoon, then progress to a regular diet, they end up having their meals in the dining room along with every-

chit-chat, then to the exchange of new interests and ideas. Their appetites improve, so does their health and their outlook, and first thing you know they're participating in games and hobbies and social events."

The bulletin board in the corridor looks like a community centre social calendar: 10:30 Church, 2:00 Bingo, 2:30 Sing Song.

There are horse shows, with people togged out in western attire; bowling parties where the ladies form into teams under catchy labels like the "Prairie Blue Belles", and St. Mary's "Sophisticates", and where "Kool Kat Cullington"

There are trips to Beacon Hill Park to watch the ships on the ocean, visits with church groups, and parties.

"We make any excuse for a party — birthdays, anniversaries, Valentine's Day, Hallowe'en — and the ladies help with preparations, and have the fun of a countdown," says Mrs. McIver.

One of the happiest events of the year is the annual December "Operation Wheelchair". Woodwards opens its store for an evening. The St. John Ambulance assist with transference to and from the hospital, and with the necessary trips to the store toilets. The Salvation Army contributes doughnuts and coffee, all so the little ladies from the Priory can do their Christmas shopping.

"We use spending money as therapy," Mrs. McIver says. "Carrying a purse, making change, the act of choosing an item, is all good mental exercise for our ladies. And they get so much joy out of being allowed to give once in a while — instead of always having to take. It really makes Christmas joyful for them."

You see the results of the Priory Method as you walk down the halls of the hospital. The wards, the beds, are empty. The patients are out just enjoying themselves, not realizing that they are being "Remotivated."

And the cost of all this? Still based on the governmental one dollar a day per person.

"Dollars won't stop a person turning into a mushroom," says Vera McIver. "But the value of tender, loving care and a lot of imagination is beyond price."

Tomorrow: "You don't need a palace": just make it practical.

Renovations also included activity and lounge spaces for visiting and carrying out meaningful interaction as well as activities of living. This decreased the social deprivation that occurred when residents had to remain in bed or languish sitting at the bedside.

Providing meaningful rather than purposeless work for residents was seen as a vital necessity for a humane life at the Priory. The goal here was to prevent life-long behaviors from becoming extinguished through lack of opportunity to exercise these abilities. She was concerned that the sight of a wheelchair automatically lowered peoples' expectations about what the residents could do. She reasoned that, within their limitations and personal preferences, they could tidy their own rooms, take care of their own toiletry, assist someone less able with their toiletry, set the table, tidy library books, and read and write for those less able. She felt that by being useful again, life would have more meaning. But individual needs and preferences had to be respected so that arts and crafts were not the only activities that were made available. To provide adequate variety and assistance it was necessary to involve the community and volunteers as well as families and friends.[39] The idea of building the Priory as a community, discussed later in this section, was another way of addressing this need.

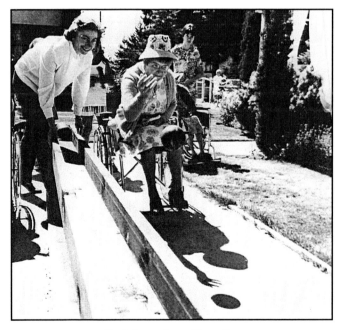

Outdoor bowling fun.

---

[39] McIver, V. (1973, February). A new environment for extended care. Proceedings of the Seminar on Extended Care. British Columbia Hospitals' Association. Richmond, BC. 40.

SAMPLE STRATEGIES THAT HUMANIZE THE LIVING SPACE

Policies	Physical Changes
• Respect for staff • Removed negative policies and procedures (the shalt nots) such as restrictive visiting hours **Staff Behavior** • Staff and residents called by first name • Staff encouraged to participate in activities e.g. staff part of festivities • Cook served meals in residents' environment • Talked to residents while walking and giving care **Example of Meaningful Activities** • Volunteering – e.g. man the reception desk, give out mail • Service e.g. projects for children • Religious e.g. setting up altar • Intellectual – e.g. discussion groups • Arts and Crafts • Group work e.g. grand parenting, tours, physical exercises • Gardening • Musical evenings and formation of a band which entered competition • Wine-making **Special Events e.g.** • Halloween Treats for children • Horse show • Annual community parade participation with a float • Pet Shows • Bowling on the lawn • Excursions • Christmas shopping spree • Knitting for refugees • Celebrating the landing on the moon	• Removed excess furniture to allow for easy wheelchair movement • Personal Possessions, Bed Throws allowed • Full spectrum lighting • Creation of nooks for friendly visiting • Use of a large table with cards and books for people to gather around • Creative use of 12-bed wards to create community and prevent isolation • Residents kitchen • Wheelchair height telephone • Created a post office run by a resident Postmistress • Shopping carts for going to the auxiliary store **Socialization Tools** • Developed conversation cue cards for the back of wheelchairs • Patients taken out of their rooms to encourage socialization • Introduced wine, pets and babies • No restrictions to visiting hours • Matching compatible room-mates and all shifts consulted • Welcomed babies and young people • Communal dining and family style mealtimes • Library and newspapers available **Activities** • Sensory stimulation and retraining • Reality Therapy • Oral History Life Review • Remotivation therapy • Reality Orientation • Milieu therapy • Music available

4. The Priory as a Community

McIver observed that the residents of the Priory were isolated from the community at large. Within the facility they were not seen and did not see themselves as being a community even though this was their living environment. Commenting on this McIver noted that:

> The residents were silent recipients; they did not participate, nor were they expected to. There was no meaningful communication... A community in order to be viable must contain certain basic balanced ingredients, such as a comfortable home, a good living environment, services, a source of work, educational opportunities, recreation and shops. A person cannot live in isolation. One has to have a sense of belonging and fellowship with others of similar interests.[40]

Community building became an essential element in the model. In normal living there is a back and forth flow between homes and the community in which they are embedded. Traditionally, hospitals have restricted this flow by using policies and procedures to close their boundaries to the world outside. McIver broke this pattern by opening up the hospital so that families, volunteers and community groups could participate in the life of residents.

There were many outings to tourist attractions made possible by utilizing families and the indispensable volunteers. A special bus was used for excursions to places such as the provincial museum, to the world-famous Butchart Gardens and for shopping tours.

Community-related activities were to have a purpose and were not to be just "make work" projects. For instance the local R.C.M.P. became involved in teaching the ladies in the correct use of their wheelchairs. It began with a driver's course given by one of the officers that included training in turning, steering, stopping and safe operation of the wheelchair. At the completion of the course the residents received a certificate acknowledging their skill. In another instance residents were involved in making Easter favors for the children of the staff. The eggs were hidden by the ladies who then watched the excited children return with their filled baskets.[41]

---

[40] McIver, V. (1999). Unpublished manuscript. p. 23.
[41] Narroway, M.D. (1974, December). Living Message. 5-7.

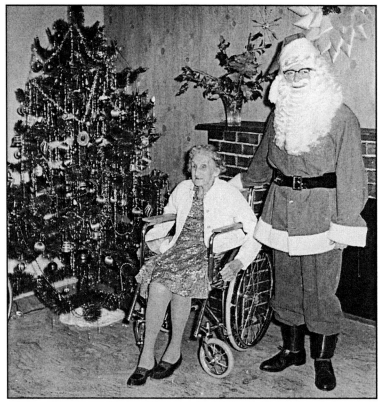

Resident enjoying Christmas festivities

Bringing in the Community

To instill pride, we bring in hairdressers, wig and makeup demonstrators, introducing the latest styles and trends. It is all fun...you should hear the giggling that goes on when one of the resident's husbands joins in the demonstrations. In the summer, there was the Priory Stampede with performing horses on the hospital grounds. You should have heard the residents, "I like the bucking one! This is just like Calgary!" The staff lends the proper atmosphere with wearing western attire. A Mutt show also has been a lot of fun. Children bring in their pets and are given prizes. You can imagine the pleasure of the residents when they are the judges and dole out the prizes. Suddenly they feel useful; they can still bring joy and pleasure to someone[42].

---

[42] McIver,V.(1973,February). A new environment for extended care. Proceedings of the Seminar on Extended Care. British Columbia Hospitals' Association. Richmond, BC. 40.

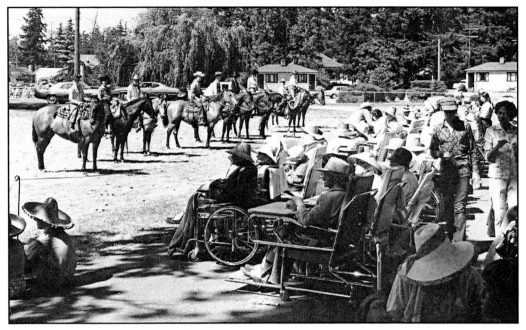

Priory stampede/rodeo.

Creating a community requires the participation of a wide range of people beyond the residents who are the focus of care.[43] All ages are required to make a viable community. Children and youth came to the Priory to share experiences with the residents, doing everything from Canadian history discussions to singing together. They were encouraged to bring their pets and kittens, puppies, bunnies, lambs and ducklings came to be cuddled by the residents. A young baby was brought in to help the women recall their days of motherhood.

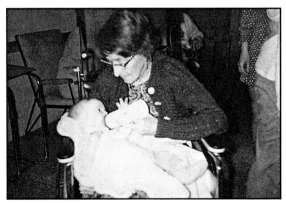

Resident feeding baby.

---

[43]   McIver, V. (1970, August). Creative Chronic Care -The Priory Method, <u>Vancouver Island Catholic News.</u> <u>2</u> (6). 8-9.

The Lions Club members poured a cement bowling alley which gave the women both competitive fun and exercise. Families were guided in communicating with their relatives, especially when Alzheimer's disease made this difficult. McIver recalls:

> We had a devoted husband who came to visit his wife daily but told us that he felt so inadequate in that all communications had ceased between them. So we gave him the simple steps of reality orientation. We showed him how to greet her, call her by name, talk about the weather, tell her that he was taking her for a ride, talk on the car ride, point out places, trees, flowers, etc, park and show her affection. At other times we advised him to bring in the newspaper and read the headlines to her and discuss them even though she is unable to respond. We invited him to turn the radio on for music. After a few days of carrying out these new interactions, this man was no longer depressed about his visits - he now had a meaningful role. (McIver, V. 2002. Personal Communication)

The creative, supportive and innovative ability of staff was a necessary ingredient in developing activities and care. Staff from all departments volunteered their time to befriend the residents and join in with activities unrelated to their departments. For instance the plant supervisor participated in the casino nights playing the role of a croupier at the roulette wheel. A secretary would leave her desk to play the piano. The housekeeper would lead hymn singing on Sunday mornings. A chef would find her way from cooking duties to dance with the residents to the tunes played by her father-in-law. A husband of one of the staff members was always in charge of barbecuing. Through acceptance and encouragement, families, friends and volunteers helped to build the community with the residents through social rehabilitation. In this way all were offered an opportunity to participate in the community of the Priory.

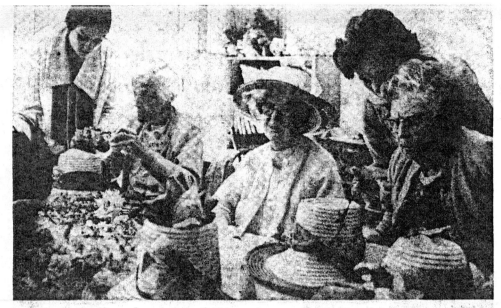

Staff members help in design and construction of Easter bonnets

Seniors Gain Fuller Lives
When Wards Lose Starch

Reproduced from The Colonist, April, 1973.

SAMPLE ACTIVITIES THAT CREATE THE PRIORY AS A COMMUNITY

- Increased contact with the community
- The Hospital within viewed as a community
- Initiated Resident Council
- Purchased a bus for outings
- Encouraged family participation – welcomed and offered hospitality and unrestricted visiting. Family members taught relevant communication strategies to help with visiting
- Encouraged volunteer participation

- Residents taken out to teas and on bus trips, shopping and outdoors
- School children invited in
- Participation in local community parades
- Use of a volunteer choir for spiritual services
- Use of community churches in providing regular services
- Family nights where families and residents celebrate together
- Service clubs invited to become involved

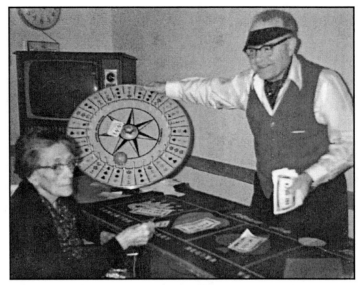

Maintenance staff involving resident in activity.

SPECIAL SITUATIONS

1. Dealing with Dementia

When McIver began her work in 1967 little was known about dementia and Alzheimer's disease. Older persons with disturbing and/or unusual behaviour were referred to as being senile. McIver disliked this word as she found it to be meaningless and demeaning. She preferred to call these more disturbed residents 'mentally impaired'. Knowledge about dementia grew slowly and as more was understood the Priory programme reflected these newer understandings. However at the beginning, the residents were initially treated in the same manner as everybody else. Because the impaired residents had no specific diagnosis, they were put into all the regular programmes and some did improve.

Looking back, McIver feels that the improvement was probably due to the fact that they were no longer neglected. An example of such improvements can be seen in the behavior of a resident who had regressed to the point where she no longer used intelligible speech. Her only verbalization had been to utter the phrase "Pi, pi". Based on the expectation that this woman was still capable of growth as a human being, she was given a kitten to hold. As she stroked it, murmuring her one phrase, the kitten began to purr. After some days of this behavior she astonished everyone by saying quite clearly "Come kitty" - these were the first words she had spoken in months.[44]

---

[44]   Narroway, M.D. (1974, December). <u>Living Message</u>. 6.

Over time, the understanding of McIver and the staff grew about the limits of the regular care programmes for residents with dementia. The well residents found their behaviour such as aggressive acts disturbing. It was decided to segregate those with the most difficult behaviors in a 12-bed ward cared for by two care aides. This was one of the earliest examples of a dementia care unit. In the center of the ward there was a kitchen table containing memory cues such as catalogues and magazines. The table acted as a place of gathering for this much smaller community. A nook with chesterfield and chairs was provided for visiting with family and friends providing a means of socialization for both the residents and their families. Many of the residents in this small ward attempted friendship in this intimate and safe environment.

As knowledge increased about dementia, McIver was able to take advantage of the environmental modifications found to be beneficial for this population. For instance, certain kinds of lighting were found to have a positive influence on behaviour and these lights were installed. Staff was permanently assigned to this ward eliminating the usual practice of rotating staff through various groupings of residents. This provided a stable and more predictable environment with caregivers who came to know their residents intimately. Here is yet another example of McIver being ahead of her time. The idea of permanent assignments in long-term care has re-surfaced in our time with the increased scientific understanding of the needs of persons with dementia from whatever cause. The residents were not confined to the unit but continued to go to the larger dining room, attend activities, and benefit from the outside environment.

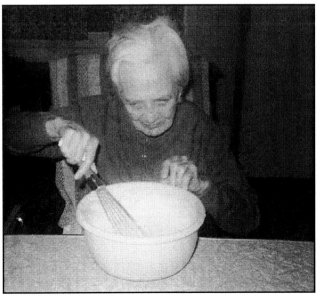

Resident enjoying being a help in the kitchen.

By 1975 Saunders had been hired as an assistant to McIver and took over an in-service role. Saunders writes about the programme of that period.[45] This programme was developed for residents who now carried the diagnosis of Organic Brain Syndrome (OBS). Care strategies were shifted from a focus on reality orientation directly, to a focus on functional change. Through the process of ego support and insight therapy geared to the resident's level of understanding, the resident was helped to deal with the anxiety generated by memory loss. Saunders suggests that even severely regressed residents were capable of learning when expectations of their abilities were realistic. Through sensory stimulation and creating an environment to make reality palatable the attempt was made to reverse the process of disengagement. Finally through life in the Priory community residents were able to exercise their remaining human functions that enhance the quality of life.

2. Hospice Care

Influenced by the work of the Hospice movement in Britain, McIver believed that the Priory had to develop a holistic approach to working with dying elders. In contrast to premature death in younger people resulting from disease, dying was seen as a natural outcome in the process of aging and an inevitable experience in the human journey. The negative effects produced by the acute care model used by most professionals appalled her. In this model pain was not well handled. Doctors and nurses conspired with families to keep patients in the dark about the reality of their situation. Care was given in an efficient, dispassionate and detached manner. Spiritual needs were to be addressed only by a priest. Contact with families was limited and difficult.[46]

However at the Priory attention was to be paid to mind and spirit as well as the body. Drawing on the work of Corbett and Hai,[47] McIver determined that "intensive caring instead of intensive care" was to be the central concept on which planning was to be based. McIver supported good pain management based on individual need and using contemporary analgesic regimes such as those found in England in the hospice movement. Excellent basic care and symptom management were not to be neglected.

But while the psychosocial environment of the Priory already in place supported staff and families, it was not enough. In her published article on the

[45] Saunders, P. (1976). Lesson 13, Section III Remotivation Therapy – What is it? Programme Manual. Unpublished. 24.
[46] McIver, V. (1980, September). A time to be born: a time to die. Canadian Nurse Journal. 76(8). 38-41.
[47] Corbett, T.L. & Lai, D. M. (1979, March). Searching for euthanatos: the hospice alternative. Hospital Progress. 60(3). 38-41, 76.

topic she went further and advocated "living experiences must be offered at this time so that the person can experience quality of life suited to his needs for as long as he can enjoy this participation."[48] In one speech she gave an example of what this might look like when she spoke in the voice of a dying person:

> If weather permits, take me outdoors, there is no reason for me to stay in my room. Going out allows me to see nature's beauties. I am sure I will appreciate them more than ever before. It will also give me a feeling of freedom and perhaps let me forget my impending death...........Suggest my family bring the family album. If you are asked to look at a picture or two, suffer a little patience, encourage me to write my autobiography or make a scrapbook of my past. These activities will give me the opportunity of telling and re-telling my story, thereby helping me.....Do not indulge me thereby creating a dependency; rather interest me in activities of daily living for as long as possible. Maintain an air of expectancy, so that I will not give in too early.[49]

Staff began by openly acknowledging death when asked about it. Residents were asked to remember Mrs. X in their prayers if her condition was deteriorating. Prayers were said at the bedside. After a death there was a short memorial during the morning activities and families were welcome to attend. Full memorial services were held for those who were alone. At one memorial service, a band was invited to provide the music. There was wine and a generous spread for all. The daughter presented each staff member with a rose. With the daughter, the life of the mother was celebrated.

IMPLEMENTING RESTORATIVE CARE

McIver's greatest challenge was to help the staff reorient their methods of practice from acute care to the Restorative Care model. In her view it took a nurse more than a year to drop the acute care biases. In addition to the programmatic activities previously listed, a number of implementing strategies were employed to assist all staff in the transition to Restorative Care.

---

[48] McIver, Vera. (1975, April). I Am a Unique Person. Speech presented at the Convention, Saskatchewan Association of Special Care Homes. Saskatoon, Sask.

[49] McIver, V. (1976, March). Cast Me Not Off In Time of My Death. Notes for a speech presented at St Joseph's School of Nursing, Victoria General Hospital. Victoria, BC. 7.

1. Resident-Centered Care Planning

McIver purchased the American Nurses Association Care Plan and modified it to meet the needs of the older residents. The comprehensive nature of the plan gave the registered nurses an opportunity to get to know their residents as persons and involved input from families, friends and doctors. Soon you heard a nurse saying, "Did you know Mrs. Jones was a pianist?" and the resident was directed toward the piano. A new database revealed many problems that the acute care nurses had not encountered before. Did the shoes, feet and toenails require attention? Was the resident really deaf or was there only a buildup of wax? Did the person wear a hearing aid and did it work? Did the resident need to see a dentist? Were relationships with family members intact? From this database the resident emerged as a person. In one instance it was discovered that hostility had developed between a son living in New York and the mother never heard from him. The staff contacted the son and the mother was overjoyed when a letter arrived from him.

2. Systematic Approach to Care

Both the multi-disciplinary health team and the support services team used a systematic approach in planning their actions. Assessment, planning, intervention and evaluation were the steps of the process. For the nurses this was one of the earliest instances where the 'nursing process' was used although it was not usually called by that name. This process promoted a careful monitoring of the physical, physiological, intellectual, social and emotional dimensions of the resident's life. Through planned interventions and a supportive environment, all residents were given the opportunity to reach and maintain their potential.

3. The Use of Prompter Cards

In order to communicate information derived from the database, prompter cards were developed. Pertinent information was transcribed onto a small introductory card that was placed in a small pouch sewn onto the back of the wheelchair. In order to initiate a conversation with the resident one would simply slip out the card and see their name, their country of origin, their family constellation and their interests. For instance, a lady had a daughter named Mary living in Vancouver and a son Tom who was a doctor in Toronto. She enjoyed classical music and knitting. "Have you heard from Tom lately?" "What are you knitting?" These were just ordinary but meaningful questions.

4. Prescribing Staff Attitudes

McIver believed that helpful staff attitudes should be individually prescribed based on an assessment of a resident's needs. This would result in everyone approaching the resident in the same way with the same expectations. For instance, a matter-of-fact attitude was used when one was trying to help a person gain independence. This was based on her belief that persons were responsible for their own behavior and must be encouraged to do all they can. The staff also had to be encouraged to do as little as possible to help in order to make the resident self-reliant.[50]

5. Permanent Shifts

Permanent shifts (working only days, evening, or nights with the same residents rather than rotating through each shift) were created for all care staff. It fostered on-going relationships that enhanced the staff's knowledge of the resident and brought about consistency in the care. The value of this is found in the words of a care aide:

> I work a permanent day shift based on a 37 1/2-hr week, and 35-day rotation. This not only suits my family life but also benefits the residents. They are more comfortable, relaxed and secure having the same person getting them up and the same for the evenings when they have the same person putting them to bed night after night. Most residents find it very hard to cope with a constant changeover of staff.[51]

6. Expanding the Notion of Team

In the mid sixties health care professionals tended to practice in isolation of each other and they each guarded their "turf." Social Workers felt that their information was so confidential that it could not be shared. Physiotherapists tended to do their work in a very separate area and would send requisitions to nursing staff to have the resident brought to the therapy room at specified periods of the day and week. It would be kept separate from the daily activities of living and there was little communication with other staff. Nurses not only did traditional nursing work but also they often had to pick up other professionals' work when they went home at the end of the day or when they were not available on evenings, nights or week-ends. Physicians were rarely on site.

[50]   McIver, V. (1974, September 6). Reactivation to Self-Feeding. Paper presented at The Priory Hospital, Victoria, BC. 3.

[51]   Williamson, F. (1978). A Psychosocial Model of Health Care: The Priory Concept - a Baseline Approach: An Environment for Long-Term Care: A Canadian Nursing Study Review. Unpublished monograph prepared as a result of a Florence Nightingale Scholarship. 42.

Non-professionals working as care aides and kitchen, housekeeping, and maintenance staff were not considered part of the team.

McIver believed that all staff needed to work as a community, visible to one another and sharing knowledge and skills to improve the well being of the residents. The staff was comprised of different types of caregivers, each with a different set of roles and activities. On a daily on-going basis residents related to the registered nurses and care aides not only by verbal communication but also through the intimate physical contact during care. Other members of the team had regular contact with the residents and with each other based on the nature of their work.

In the Priory Model the membership on the team was enlarged and role overlap was supported amongst all staff. Flexibility in job functions whenever it was of benefit to the resident was the order of the day. Modeled after the home setting, nursing staff would assist in the dining room with toast making or wipe up a spill from the floor. Housekeeping, maintenance and kitchen staff were active participants in the team becoming personally involved in resident care. They encouraged residents, interacted with them, helped them at mealtimes and joined in with their activities. The cook's therapeutic role in being sensitive to the psychological component as it relates to food was highlighted. Good nutritional health hinged on well-balanced and tasty meals served in an attractive environment. Having the cook serve the meals ensured immediate feedback on the residents' response to meals. Families were also members of the team and provided insight into the resident's strengths and any liabilities they may possess. Their participation in the team supported the maintenance of the resident's role within the family and further normalized the life of the resident.[52]

A concrete example of multidisciplinary work can be drawn from the area of rehabilitation. The physiotherapist was seen as the resource person to teach the skills of physical rehabilitation to staff, residents and family. For example, a resident may be taught how to transfer but this needed to be followed through by all caregivers and staff, especially those closest to the resident. It was the registered nurse who coordinated and incorporated the expertise of all disciplines into a dynamic care plan because nursing was present 24 hours a day, seven days a week.[53]

---

[52]   Williamson, F. (1978). A Psychosocial Model of Health Care: The Priory Concept - a Baseline Approach: An Environment for Long-Term Care: A Canadian Nursing Study Review. Unpublished monograph prepared as a result of a Florence Nightingale Scholarship. 52.

[53]   Saunders, P. (1976). Lesson 12, Section IV: Specific Implementation of Concepts. Programme Manual. Unpublished. 17.

7. Resident-focused Conferences, Councils and Family Meetings

Regularly scheduled resident conferences, which included the family and the team, were seen as essential to goal setting. This was where the needs, problems, likes and dislikes as well as past rituals could be brought to light. The conferences also focused on establishing the attitudinal approach to be used with the resident. All staff including housekeepers, maintenance and dietary were included as part of the team and became promoters of Restorative Care.

In the new model of care residents were supported to take initiative in planning their own recreational and social activities. In order to provide opportunity for the residents to be self-directing Resident Councils were established.[54] Councils were under the direction of the Social Worker and met informally appointing their own executive. They made recommendations on a variety of issues that were then forwarded to Administration for approval.[55]

Family input was essential to the team approach as it unfolded in the Priory Method. Family nights were introduced to foster this discussion. Families and staff spent an evening together on a regular basis during which time serious discussions about care were interspersed with lighter conversation and activities. Small groups were formed once topics were brought forth and solutions were sought.

McIver's unique role in the post-1967 Priory organization facilitated the implementation of Restorative Care practice. She became both the senior clinical nurse and the manager of all patient care and support services. This position simplified her work as it was through this position that she could introduce the new clinical approaches discussed in this chapter *and* support them with the appropriate management infrastructure discussed in chapter 4. [56]

---

[54] McIver, V. (1974, July). Notes for Presentation to the Staff of Ponoka Long-term Care Facility. Ponoka, Alberta.

[55] Williamson. Frank. (1978). A Psychosocial Model of Health Care: The Priory Concept - a Baseline Approach: An Environment for Long-Term Care: A Canadian Nursing Study Review. Unpublished monograph prepared as a result of a Florence Nightingale Scholarship. 50.

[56] Even in to-day's terms, the scope of this kind of role is an unusual arrangement but it gave her the freedom to make sweeping innovations.

chapter 4

Creating an Organizational Environment for Restorative Care

McIver's involvement with the Canadian Hospital Association Programme "Hospital Organization and Its Management" introduced management and staff to the literature of Argyris, Likert, and Hertzberg.[57] The humanistic view of management put forth by these authors was influential in encouraging McIver and her administrator to change. McIver learned from her studies that in order to change the way in which residents and their families were cared for and the manner in which staff worked, the total environment had to undergo change. She came to know that:

> The environment to be therapeutic must have the climate that radiates confidence, trust, and commitment to a person centered program. Developing a healing environment could not be left to happenstance. It had to be based on knowledge and sound humanistic principles of management, which respect the individuality of each person.[58]

In this chapter we consider the management infrastructure which supported the care practices and which was put in place simultaneously with the care programmes. We begin with the guiding ideas that directed the changes. We follow with the three critical areas of structural/functional change which supported the Priory Method: a movement to a hotel services orientation for the support services; the introduction of innovative roles; and policies developed for a new order. We conclude with a discussion of the impact of such a major transition and some of the approaches used to facilitate the shift. On page 54, **Figure 4** shows the changes introduced by McIver transplanted onto the Restorative Care tree used by her as a metaphor.

---

[57] Argyris.C. (1957). <u>Personality and Organization</u>. New York:Harper and Row; Likert R. (1967). <u>Human Organization</u>. Toronto:McGraw Hill; Hertzberg. H. (1966). <u>Work and the Nature of Man</u>. Montreal: Crowell Press. As cited in McIver. V. (1979, November). Organization of integrated extended care facilities. <u>Dimensions in Health Care</u>. 1.

[58] McIver, V. (1999). Unpublished manuscript.

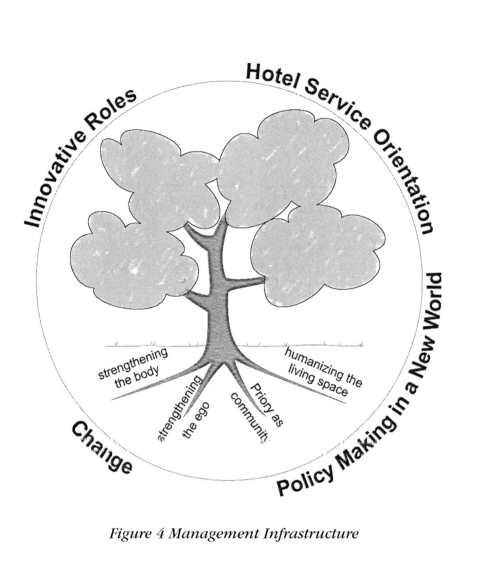

Figure 4 Management Infrastructure

GUIDING IDEAS FOR THE INFRASTRUCTURE AT THE PRIORY[59]

The philosophy was the cornerstone upon which the system was to be built (see page 21). The literature guided McIver to involve workers in their jobs through job enlargement, job enrichment and provision of opportunities for personal expression and growth including their involvement in decision-making. In the new Priory organization the following strategies were used to operationalize these ideas.

---

[59]   McIver, V. (1977, July). <u>Humanizing the Workplace</u>. Unpublished paper.

- Unnecessary tasks were removed to allow the role occupant to provide the care for which they had been educated. For instance a unit coordinator position (discussed on page 58) was introduced to relieve nurses of most non-professional and administrative duties and this allowed them to fully practice their nursing skills in applying the philosophy.
- Staff was given the freedom to communicate both horizontally and diagonally as well as vertically in order to gather data and communicate more effectively.
- Leadership and innovative abilities were fostered and persons were expected to assume responsibility for decision-making consistent with the position they held. For example, the registered nurse team leader was held accountable for his/her actions without a constant overview by a supervisor. The immediate supervisor was seen not only as an evaluator but also as a resource person and a colleague. This same trust was given to all staff including the cook and the housekeeper.
- The span of control of a manager was broad and this reduced the need for executives and department heads. In this regard McIver was influenced by the writings of Argyris who believed that a small span of control fostered a master-servant relationship and this ran counter to the philosophy.
- A departmental structure was eschewed as non-nursing professionals were added to the team. By removing the administrative and non-professional duties necessary in running a department, the professional practitioners were on the unit practicing on behalf of the residents. A genuine team approach was facilitated because all met on common ground as they shared the same space and concerns.
- Roles were blurred between workers as they became involved with each other and with all the aspects concerning the resident.

THE CHANGE TO A HOTEL SERVICES ORIENTATION

In the 1960's, hospitals in the acute care sector had support services that served to maintain an acute-crisis, illness-oriented model. McIver viewed such services as inappropriate for long-term care. Residents "lived" at the Priory for an extended period of time and it was considered to be their "home." She believed that the new philosophy and Restorative Care model required something closer to the services offered by hotels and she adopted this term as she found it discussed in the literature of that time.

Under the hotel services rubric new positions were created and traditional roles altered to bring them into line with the philosophy. Laundry, plant services and housekeeping were still required but were seen to focus on the needs of the residents in their home. Home-like bed linens, blankets, bedspreads along with housekeeping tasks that pertained more to the day-to-day upkeep of a home were the priority for these services. Residents no longer dressed in hospital attire (hospital gown and slippers) but wore their own personal clothing such as dresses and shoes. A new position referred to by McIver as 'Wardrobe Mistress' was established to help residents and families buy clothes that would then be adjusted as required for individual needs. A seamstress was now also required as special care and attention for personal clothing was needed.

Meals were served through dining room services rather than being based in a traditional hospital kitchen where food was sent to patients on trays. McIver believed that kitchen staff needed to have face-to-face contact with the residents and residents needed to see and smell the food they were being served. The cook needed to have immediate feedback on the responses of the residents. Thus the cook, dressed in chef's attire, served the food in the dining room from hot bulk food containers.

Table 2 (on page 57) compares the support services found in the acute care hospital of the late sixties with the model instituted by McIver for the Priory.

Innovative Roles

Breaking with tradition and using creative titles to reflect the changing management structure, McIver created new staff roles as well as re-configuring traditional roles.[60] The new positions gave fresh meaning to the work and to the relationships with residents and between staff members. These roles supported the staff and management in the implementation of the new care programmes and the home-like atmosphere designed for the residents. The structure eliminated the superior-subordinate staff relationships and focused instead on individuals' self discipline and responsibility to carry out their tasks. The changes are documented below.

1. Hospital Services Director

The first change was in the Nursing Director's title and function. The position of Director of Nursing Services was eliminated and the Nursing Services Department was incorporated under the leadership of a new position, Hospital Services Director. This was the role filled by McIver who reported directly to

---

[60] McIver, V. (1972, November). <u>Staffing.</u> Paper given to The Registered Nurses Association Of British Columbia. Vancouver, BC.

Table 2

Comparison of Support Services
Acute Care and St. Mary's Priory

	ACUTE CARE HOSPITAL MODEL SUPPORT SERVICES	ST MARY'S PRIORY HOTEL SERVICES
Focus	• episodic illness (surgical, medical) & emergencies, • functional and efficient environment • patients on bed rest , dependency, leading to incapacity, total care • areas departmentalized/centralized • services delivered to the patient by disease entities	• residential care, home environment, hotel orientation • long stay residents with little turnover • focus on self-care/activities of daily living • Not departmentalized • service delivered to resident based on need
Laundry Department	• no reusable supplies so heavy demand on this service • primarily for bed linens and patient hospital gowns and baby diapers as well as specialized departments e.g. operating room, Emergency, Delivery room	• homelike bed linens, blankets and spreads • residents' personal clothing and personal bed coverings • wardrobe mistress and seamstress to take care of resident clothing
Central supply Room	• no disposable items – reusable service only • to clean, wrap, sterilize and distribute equipment and supplies to the units & special services	• basic supplies cared for at the unit level • minimal equipment e.g. oxygen sphygmomanometer, non-disposable basic dressing trays & catheter sets, small unit sterilizer
Dietary & Food Services	• large centralized kitchens with food sent on bulk order to units in heated trolleys • trays assembled on the unit by dietary aides and delivered by nurses • variety of therapeutic diets managed by dietitian • wards have minimal access to food and drink	• meal and dining room services • family style dining • cooks and food service workers interact directly with residents • special food events (Birthdays, picnics • readily available snacks and drinks on unit with self serve in residents' kitchen and dining room
Plant Services	• focus on buildings and grounds – boilers/heating/water supply and incinerator • patient use not a focus • highly specialized equipment e.g. respirators, OR machines, iron lungs, suction machines, oxygen tanks	• unit-based and homelike in approach • focus on wheelchairs, beds, commodes • staff have direct involvement with residents acting as volunteers, support workers • directly related to maintaining homelike atmosphere in gardens and buildings for resident & family use
House-keeping	• orientation on reducing transfer of infection, terminal cleaning of units • cleaning of floors/walls/bed pans/urinals/washbasins/water jugs • heavy equipment used for cleaning and polishing floors	• home-like jobs e.g. floor washing, dusting, bathroom hygiene • lighter equipment for manual washing and damp dusting

the Administrator. The role expanded beyond nursing to include all health services (nursing, pharmacy, social work, physiotherapy, and health records). As well,
the responsibilities now embraced the hotel functions identified on page 56
and were a good example of role augmentation. This enabled integration of all
care and support services under one manager. Common philosophies and goals
could now more readily be implemented with this integration.

In addition to the administrative functions, McIver as the Hospital Services
Director, assumed the clinical practice leadership role referred to earlier. The
additional clinical functions included overseeing the development, implementation, monitoring and evaluation of all Restorative Care programmes. She organized meetings with staff to develop standards and intervention protocols
for care. She was visible on the unit where care was taking place, acting as role
model and teacher as she led the implementation of the programme.

2. Unit Coordinator

The next major role change was the introduction of a new role titled Unit
Coordinator. This role occupant had several responsibilities that included supervising all hotel services at the unit level, acting as a link between the health
and hotel services and providing administrative support to nursing.

The Unit Coordinator was responsible for hotel services on the unit such as
wardrobe, laundry, linen services, food services, plant services, and housekeeping. Staffing responsibilities including scheduling, health records, admissions,
discharges and acquiring unit supplies were an integral part of the administrative support provided on the nursing unit. Many of these administrative support functions represented "non nursing" activities that previously had been
carried out by nurses preventing them from fulfilling their nursing care functions. The transfer of the non-nursing activities from nurses to the unit coordinator freed the registered nurses from these chores. Now they were able to
optimize their professional roles as clinical coordinators, care providers and
teachers, roles that were essential for the successful implementation of the
new care programmes. The identification of these "non-nursing" functions was
clearly a very insightful way of reorganizing the work of the professional registered nurse in the mid-sixties.[61] A Service Aide assisted the Unit Coordinator.
Initially the role was designed to assist both the Unit Coordinator and the health
care team. However by 1975 this aide became a full-time assistant to the Unit
Coordinator and replaced the Unit Coordinator during vacation time.

---

[61] Even in 2001 the issue of non-nursing work was still a problem as highlighted in the
      demands of the British Columbia Nurses Union. BCNU demands changes to nonnursing
      work and overtime abuse, Times-Colonist, Victoria, BC (2001, May).

A Place in the Family

The Priory has been my work-home since 1976 when I began at the Little Hospital as a cook/housekeeper. My early days were spent working with Support Services. In 1977 I was excited to transfer to the House of Peace (Priory Hospital) to work as a Service Aide assisting the Unit Coordinator and the Professional Services Coordinator. My next move was to the Administration Building to work on the Payroll and finally I moved to the Timekeeping Office. During the 1970's I took the in-house nurses' aide course and in 1989 when my children were grown I enrolled in the nursing program at the community college. Since that time I have been a Care Coordinator (see below) on the evening shift on the Priory site.

In the seventies the Priory Hospital seemed so small compared to today and it was truly a family. The residents were more capable and more involved in those days and they were the center of the Priory. We, the staff, all lived in this small community of Colwood and were neighbors so the habit of helping each other was natural for us. If there was a tea for the residents our children would stop in after school and they were always welcome at the home. The nuns had set a warm tone and it seemed to permeate all our work. There was never any sense of someone being the 'boss' because we all helped out with whatever had to be done. Our staff cohesiveness was cemented by the regular social events such as potlucks and dances at the Colwood Hall and no one would dream of missing an event.

My job as a Service Aide was very busy. It seemed to me that we were entertaining most of the time. We had so many visitors coming either to visit with their family or to see the Priory Method in operation. I spent much of my time arranging luncheons and teas. The teas were quite 'classy' as we used special china and the residents would help in whatever way they could. I was also very involved with staffing which in those days was a very satisfying job and I loved it. It was a real challenge to make sure that we had each shift adequately staffed and that the staff were happy. We knew all the individual needs of the staff as when, for instance, their baby needed to sleep and they could leave to come to work. We would work around their schedule and the staff would do anything to come in when we needed them. If someone would come but didn't have a car I would go to get them and someone else would drive them home. We had a fairly active union but there were few grievances and things worked in a very cooperative way.

I reflect back on those days and realize how much fun we had as well as having a sense of satisfaction about what we were doing.

Interview with Helen Dyer RN December, 2002

3. New Nursing Roles

Supervisory positions that had been carried out by the Nuns who were registered nurses were deleted. In their place two new nursing positions, *Professional Services Coordinator* and *Care Coordinator* were created.

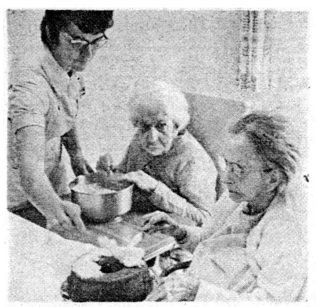

Nurse Sally Surette, Mrs. Millicent Sanders and
Mrs. Dorothy Carnie . . . getting ready for a party.

3.1 The **Professional Services Coordinator** was a registered nurse who coordinated the work of all health care disciplines and was responsible for the health care of 70-90 residents housed on one nursing unit. The responsibilities were:

- Facilitating the nursing teams work through leadership, planning, and innovation
- Coordinating, implementing and evaluating all professional disciplines
- Coordinating and evaluating other outside health care services such as dentistry, podiatry, laboratory, and x-ray
- Working in partnership with the Unit Coordinator for hotel services and non-nursing activities and
- Supervising and working with the Volunteer Coordinator (see Chapter 5) to ensure the utilization and supervision of volunteers by health care staff.[62]

---

[62] Juan de Fuca Hospitals. (1977). Educational Manual. Victoria, BC. Unpublished.

THE EXPERIENCE OF A PROFESSIONAL SERVICES COORDINATOR

*In 1977 I began working as the **Professional Services Coordinator (PSC)** at the Richmond hospital, one of the facilities which had recently come under the direction of Vera McIver. I brought to my role 11 years of nursing experience, most of it in the field of mental health. I found the role a satisfying but unusual one. In mental health I had been a Head Nurse but as a PSC I was a Head Nurse Plus Plus.*

I was the 'boss' with a lot of responsibility, some of which was new for me. Under my wing I had 75 residents and the nursing staff. Other health professionals– a social worker, physiotherapist, reactivation assistant, volunteer coordinator, pharmacist and physician – were on my team. I worked in a partnership with all the staff rather than in a traditional tiered relationship. We communicated often and there was no problem if our roles overlapped from time to time. For instance both the Social Worker and myself knew and supported the families. The Social Worker could be found moving residents in their wheelchairs and I was often involved with direct nursing care.

As a manager I was not office-bound but rather I was out on the unit with residents and staff most of the time. In this way I got to know people very well and we developed long-term relationships. I was able to do this because of the presence of the Unit Coordinator. This person was my equal and took over the 'running of the house' as McIver called it as well as the staffing. Thus I was freed to do my essential task of upholding the standards for quality care using the Priory Method.

I also interviewed and hired my own staff rather than having them assigned from the distant Nursing Office. I knew what I was looking for and after hiring I had a real commitment to that staff person. This worked both ways because they had also chosen to work with me.

Some of my best memories are of Christmas Day. The families joined us for dinner if they could. A lot of the staff came in to serve the food even if it was their day off. Throughout the year the relationships between families and the staff were very close and Christmas was no exception.

One of my biggest challenges was helping staff master the Priory Method. This required major changes for those who were educated in acute care or who had their major experience in custodial care. Building an esprit de corps was hard work but McIver helped me. She was very visible on the unit and I learned from her every visit. She talked and taught – about wellness messages and skin care and shared roles and giving people dignity – whatever was needed to move us forward in creating a home for the older people.

Interview with Margo Hughes RN BScN MEd December, 2002

3.2 The **Care Coordinator** position changed the registered nurse's priorities from being a mini nurse-administrator to that of a clinical and teaching professional nurse. This was a significant role change as it enhanced the role of the nurse in the extended care setting. In addition to providing professional nursing care when appropriate, the Care Coordinator was a team leader on her shift. This involved coordinating and supervising the care for a group of residents (30-37) who were being primarily cared for by non-professional aides. These positions were scheduled on permanent 8-hour shifts for days, evenings or nights and staff did not rotate through each shift. With this role change and with the advent of the Unit Coordinator, the nurse had more time for residents. This required a major adjustment for the registered nurse as she moved away from directing the care from the nursing station to working directly with the residents in planning, monitoring, coordinating and evaluating care.[63] Through lectures, team conferences and resident assessments, the Care Coordinator became more informed and knowledgeable about how to carry out her new role.

> ## WORKING WITH RESTORATIVE CARE
> ## THE CHALLENGE OF CHANGE
>
> *I began my role of Care Coordinator in 1977; ten years after McIver began her work. Like many of my peers, I brought to this practice, years of nursing experience in acute care hospitals. I worked on emergency, surgical and neurological units as well as having teaching experience in orthopaedics. During my work in those settings, I noticed I was continually drawn to older patients. This interest finally led me to seek a position in a long-term care hospital.*
>
> *Learning to draw information from social histories and seeing the resident as a 'whole' person, presented me with the first of many new challenges. In acute care, I tended to focus on the patient's presenting problem and once that was solved, they would exit the system and I would see them no more. Now I had to learn to think of the residents as people with whom I would have a life-long relationship. I came to know these individuals as people who were 'bigger' than their chronic illness. I recall one lady with a stroke who had once worked with preparing sterile supplies. How was this lady to find a purpose in life in her new state of being in an institution? She had only one good hand but she and I would wrap the needed supplies together making the two needed hands. This lady had the opportunity to teach me and I had a chance to*

[63] McIver. V. (1971). The Extended Role of the Registered Nurse in Extended Care. Unpublished paper. 1-5.

honor her knowledge - such was the Priory Method. I helped another resident to plan her Christmas gift list and then to help her wrap her gifts after the volunteers had taken her shopping. I knew this resident's family as intimately as my own because that was the role of nursing in this setting.

I worried if a resident was transferred to acute care where she or he might be seen primarily as a senile older person, which was often a label attached to the elderly in those days. I visited residents and talked with the nurses in acute care in an attempt to reverse this stereotypical view.

I was awakened to the individual's ability to be self-directing in care. There was a 99-year-old man who didn't want to walk but the orders read that he must be ambulated. The nurses' argued for choice – his right to decide.

My relationship to physicians changed. Some doctors thought I must have had problems in acute care and that was why I had come to long-term care. Interestingly, this view shifted over time, as we grew to respect each other's contributions, as part of a larger team, in meeting residents' needs.

Relationships with families became more comprehensive and meaningful partner-ships. Often families who had a member with dementia needed my guidance as much as did the resident. I, along with my colleagues, was anxious to embrace the tenants of the Priory method in communicating effectively with residents suffering dementia. On the other hand, my communication skills with alert residents were also sharpened as they taught me how to shape and modify my questions. I recall asking one resident who was reading a book, if it was a good book, to which the resident replied that she wouldn't be reading it if it weren't. Lesson learned – don't ask rhetorical questions!

I can remember every resident to this day. I learned I had the capacity to love them in spite of their dementia. I have retained my allegiance to what I now call gerontological nursing and I, like many others, have become a certified gerontological nurse.

Interview with Irene Harris, RN, BScN December, 2002

3.3 In 1970 the role of **Medication Nurse** was instituted. This nurse worked on the day shift, and the first 4 hours of the evening shift. The role was estab-lished so that the Care Coordinator would no longer be occupied in the single time-absorbing task of giving medications and could focus on other aspects of resident care. The Medication Nurse was responsible for all medication-related activities appropriate for a registered nurse during her work shift. She was a participant in the resident assessment conferences with other team members and worked closely with the Care Coordinator in planning care.

4. Other Health Care Roles

New roles that supported the organization's focus on health rather than illness were established by 1970. An **Activity Coordinator** assisted by a part-time **Service Aide** was responsible for planning and guiding the implementation of purposeful activities in recreation, leisure and daily living both for individuals and for groups of residents. This was done in partnership with the nursing staff.[64]

McIver created a **Social Services Coordinator** position to be filled by a Social Worker. This was the first such position in extended care in British Columbia. She reported to the Professional Services Coordinator and was primarily concerned with the effects of long-term illness and increasing disability on the resident and /or family's health.[65] As a way of supporting the implementation of the Restorative Care programme and maximizing the potential of each resident, the Social Service Coordinator had four major responsibilities:

- arranging the admissions
- obtaining a social history and participating in the development monitoring, and evaluation of a unified plan of care for the residents and families
- creating resident and family councils as a way to facilitate resident opportunity for being self-directed and having input into the life of the community of the facility and
- guiding and referring residents and families to other community resources with such matters as pensions, wills and other legal issues.

In addressing why the Social Services Coordinator reported to the Professional Services Coordinator rather than creating a Social Work Department, McIver noted that:

> It was only natural when I hired a social worker; she would not be operating a department but would be responsible to the Professional Services Coordinator so as to maintain a flat organization. We did not want to introduce a bureaucratic organization that would stifle, or curb the talent and initiatives of those who wanted to contribute in a meaningful way. Another reason we had Social Workers and subsequent paramedical disciplines under the direction of the Professional Services Coordinator was to prevent fragmentation of care.[66]

---

[64] Williamson, F. (1978). <u>A Psychosocial Model of Health Care: The Priory Concept - a Baseline Approach: An Environment for Long-Term Care: A Canadian Nursing Study Review.</u> Unpublished monograph prepared as a result of a Florence Nightingale Scholarship. 40.

[65] McIver, V. (1970). <u>How the social worker can fit into our picture</u>. Unpublished paper.

[66] McIver, V. (1999). Unpublished manuscript. 82.

The 1970 organizational structure, which included the new roles that McIver introduced, is shown in **Figure 5** on page 66. The relationships between the various staff positions are also depicted. The position of Maintenance Supervisor on this chart was a role that focused on the 'big plant' – heating, lighting, and ventilation. Unit maintenance was filled by a worker that McIver referred to as Mr. Fix-it, who looked after unit details such as wheelchairs. The Comptroller had a single function, that of managing the finances for the hospital. This freed McIver from working with budget details although she was kept informed of the financial picture. It is significant that the Priory Method of care reduced the overall costs of care when compared to other extended care units.

5. Emerging Job Descriptions

The organizational changes made by McIver in role definition and expectations led to role overlap, a consequence she desired.[67] Flexibility in role definition whenever it was of benefit to the resident was a key premise of the Priory Method. As in the home setting, nursing staff would assist in setting up the dining room, make toast and wipe a spill off the floor. Housekeeping, maintenance and kitchen staff were personally involved in encouraging residents, interacting with them, joining in with their activities and helping at mealtimes. Job descriptions were not written in stone and the union did not express any concern about the role overlap.

The initial work on the Restorative Care Tree (see Chapter 2) had provided McIver and her colleagues with a way of looking at the residents' needs. Now this same tree became an organizing framework for a generic job description that matched roles to these needs. Role expectations for caregivers were listed under the headings of the roots of the tree as shown in **Table 3** (on page 67).

POLICY MAKING IN A NEW WORLD

In the light of all the changes that McIver implemented, she saw that acute care policies that focused on illness, dependency and life- prolonging technologies were not suitable for extended care.[68] She decided to develop a new policy and procedure manual focused specifically on extended care. The philosophy was used as a template or screen through which new materials were reviewed in order to ensure consistency with the values implicit in the philosophy and model of care. She wrote:

---

[67]   McIver, V. (1977, July). <u>Humanizing the Work Space</u>. Unpublished paper. 1-5.
[68]   McIver, V. (1974, Oct 1). <u>Policies Were Meant To Be Broken</u>. Notes for a speech presented at the You and Long-term Care Conference. Geneva Park, Lake Couchiching, Ontario.

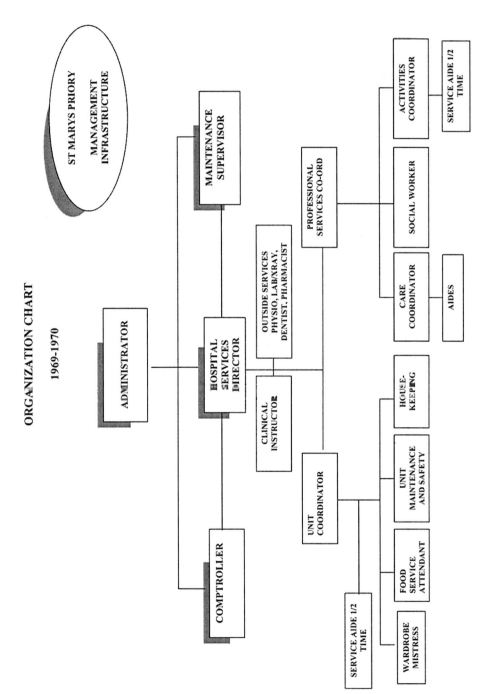

Figure 5

ORGANIZATION CHART

1969-1970

ST MARYS PRIORY
MANAGEMENT
INFRASTRUCTURE

ADMINISTRATOR

COMPTROLLER

MAINTENANCE SUPERVISOR

HOSPITAL SERVICES DIRECTOR

OUTSIDE SERVICES PHYSIO, LAB/XRAY, DENTIST, PHARMACIST

CLINICAL INSTRUCTOR

PROFESSIONAL SERVICES CO-ORD

ACTIVITIES COORDINATOR

SERVICE AIDE 1/2 TIME

SOCIAL WORKER

CARE COORDINATOR

AIDES

UNIT COORDINATOR

HOUSE-KEEPING

UNIT MAINTENANCE AND SAFETY

FOOD SERVICE ATTENDANT

WARDROBE MISTRESS

SERVICE AIDE 1/2 TIME

Table 3
Role Expectactions for Persons Providing Restorative Care [69]

Types of Care by Roots of the Tree	Role Expectations
Physiological Care	• Along with good body care, the nurse will focus on prevention to stem deterioration and rehabilitation to restore mobility • Staff will help residents re-learn the activities of daily living, e.g. feeding, dressing, grooming, and bowel and bladder control • Staff will use good body mechanics and safe techniques of lifting, transferring and body positioning to protect residents and themselves
Social Care	Staff will provide care to the resident which includes: • provision for involvement of the family, friends and the community • encouraging visitors including children • reintroducing residents to their former life style, taking into consideration culture, education, occupation and religious affiliation • avoiding unnecessary restrictions • integrating self, staff as a whole, residents' families, friends and volunteers into the social fabric of the Priory community, as well as the community at large
Spiritual Care	Staff will provide care to the resident which includes: • recognition of the role religion plays in the life of the resident, be it Christian or non-Christian sources of faith, strength and hope • working with clergy to provide spiritual support in prayer and consolation in providing hospice care to assist the resident in accepting death with grace and dignity • assisting residents in obtaining legal aid to settle affairs • providing adequate pain and comfort care • discontinuing needless monitoring • not hiding dying and death from other residents and asking for their assistance in prayer and visits • holding a memorial service with residents and family if they wish to be present • supporting family during grieving
Psychological Care	Staff will provide care to the resident which includes: • making an effort to maintain or restore the resident's identity, and foster self-reliance and confidence in self by nurturing their ego resources • encouraging personal possessions • helping residents initiate the need to be needed through small acts for others • giving emotional support and allowing residents the freedom to exercise initiatives in planning whenever possible • liberally using ego enhancers such as sincere praise and flattery, assurance, encouragement and acceptance • adding incentives for living through purposeful activities and initiating self-motivational projects to foster a feeling of self-esteem

[69] Adapted from McIver, V. (1999). Unpublished manuscript. 41-42

> The foundation stone is a central philosophy, which expresses the collective values of professionals and non-professionals within the institution. Each plan, policy or procedure is passed through this mass of stated values and beliefs, subjected to scrutiny of scientific background and eventually becomes filtered so that the action reflects the philosophy.[70]

Some of the new policies changed the daily schedules for residents to resemble those at home, such as later breakfast (moved from 7:30 AM to 8:30 AM), baths in the evening, and afternoon tea times and late evening snacks. Of major importance to McIver was a new policy that liberalized the visiting hours. Family and friends were encouraged and invited to participate in the life of loved ones in the facility at a time convenient to them. They also became involved in taking residents to participate in community life such as the symphony, ferry rides, visiting relatives and swimming.

Policies that changed the roles of the various health disciplines and support service workers improved the utilization of the human resources within the organization. All the role changes supported a focus on the needs of the elderly resident, not on the needs of the professional. For example the primary role of the pharmacist became clinical rather than the dispensing of drugs. Physiotherapists carried out their therapy as an activity in the resident's room or with groups of residents rather than in a remote office to which the resident had to be taken. The Unit Coordinator picked up the non-nursing duties so that the nurses could focus on the resident.

IMPLEMENTING CHANGE

It was not an easy transition for the staff to bring about these role and care-giving changes. McIver recalls the resistance; some nurse quit and some worked against administration and attempted to influence the others. For McIver, the residents were of prime concern so the organizational development continued towards fulfilling her vision in spite of the resistance. To do so McIver involved the union leadership by keeping them informed and up to date with all plans.

A major challenge was to find nursing staff who were eager to learn and work with the new philosophy. It was McIver's view that an all registered nurse staff was not required. She worked with the community college to provide an educational programme for Resident Care Attendants (often called care aides in other settings). She provided one of her degree-prepared registered nurses to teach the course and the Priory was used as their clinical education setting.

---

[70] McIver, V. (1978, March). Freedom to be: A new approach to quality care for the aged: Part two: The Priory Method. <u>Canadian Nurse Journal</u>. <u>74</u>(3). 24.

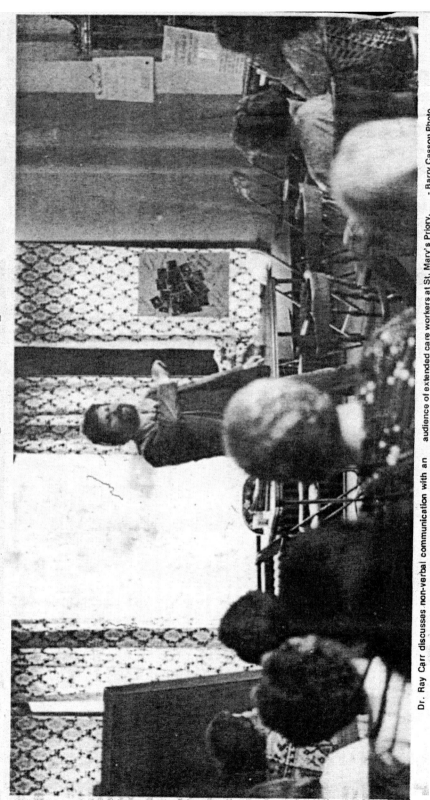

THE VICTORIAN — MONDAY, APRIL 29, 1974

Workshop explores ways to improve extended care

Dr. Ray Carr discusses non-verbal communication with an audience of extended care workers at St. Mary's Priory.   - Barry Casson Photo

This approach not only served McIver's needs but also allowed her to influence the educational curriculum and bring the needs of older people to the attention of educators.

She realized that given the significant changes to staff roles and care delivery, staff education needed to be valued and viewed as a high priority. She believed that each staff member had the potential for growth and a Programme Coordinator was hired to:

- Develop and implement an orientation and regular in-service education programmes
- Develop staff education committees to focus on specific education needs of staff and arrange for education sessions and
- Develop a reference library on each unit, readily accessible to all staff.

An education budget was created and processes for assisting staff to attend conferences and seminars were developed. Policies for staff development and education were established.[71] With education and the visible positive results of the change in the residents, staff resistance changed to one of support and progress was made in improving care and meeting the goals.

McIver became politically active in a small "p" sense. Her letters to politicians documenting real situations led to a change in facility discharge criteria. People who showed improvement with remotivation programmes and who were admitted to a facility prior to the government involvement in long term care, were no longer discharged to a facility offering less care. They could remain in their "facility home" for as long as they lived. . She wrote several papers to government and the Registered Nurses Association of British Columbia to substantiate the level of care required for residents in extended care.[72]

The press became her ally when she found the way to show the benefits of the Priory Method to the reading public of the newspapers. In this monograph we have used a number of photographs from these newpaper articles. At the official Priory opening when rennovations were complete, she had journalist-photographers take pictures of the empty beds which had been occupied only 6 months prior under custodial care. The accompanying newspaper article showed that the Priory residents were all up and active.

McIver was challenging the usual way of doing things and this was not always comfortable for others or successful. In her view one of her greatest problems was dealing with the government bureaucracy. For instance she took

---

71 Williamson, F. (1978). A Psychosocial Model of Health Care:The Priory Concept - a Baseline Approach: An Environment for Long-Term Care: A Canadian Nursing Study Review. Unpublished monograph prepared as a result of a Florence Nightingale Scholarship. 67-71.

72 McIver, V. (1971). Workload-Staff requirements. Unpublished paper.

particular exception to the Ministry Blue Design Guide for architectural planning. While it was reported to be for extended care facilities it was based on the needs of acute care hospital patients and ignored the needs of residents in long term care facilities. She wanted it changed. As chair of a committee of the Registered Nurses Association of British Columbia she brought a government architect to the table and gained his support for her newer ideas. While this approach put the contemporary ideas into the general architectural community, it did not convince everyone and with some building projects underway, any revision of the Guide was stopped. On another occasion she recalls that she had been invited to speak to physicians about the Priory Method. The invitation was withdrawn and her recollection was that the government consultant had advised that her talk be cancelled. As well her articles were no longer published in the BCHIS publication. These examples show that every change agent must be prepared to meet some resistance as they challenge the status quo about the way to do business and they speak to McIver's courage in meeting this resistance.

McIver understood that caring for older people was more than creating a relevant model of care and an infrastructure which would support that care. By 1978 she was able to write:

> A positive philosophy, scientific evidence, imaginative planning of the environment – these are all necessary for the rehabilitation of the aged. But there is one modification, the least expensive of all, that assumes an importance above the others because its absence is felt most acutely by the residents. That ingredient is loving, expressed through therapeutic attitudes, such as listening, smiling, talking and touching.[73]

---

[73] McIver, V. (1978, March). Freedom to be: A new approach to quality care for the aged: Part two: The Priory Method. Canadian Nurse Journal. 74(3). 25.

chapter 5

Moving Forward

The Priory Method was a dynamic model that changed over time as a result of both internal and external factors. Evaluations from a variety of sources reinforced some ideas and modified others. The organization expanded and new staff came on board, many of whom were unfamiliar with the Priory Method. McIver retired in 1979 but the ideas were never completely lost. As we entered the new millennium a new facility, Heritage Woods, emerged on the Priory site embodying many of the ideas that McIver had espoused. In this chapter we show the evolution of the model and its subsequent growth over time. First we discuss the success of the Priory Method. We move on to document how the organization expanded towards the end of McIver's tenure and the subsequent evolution of the Priory Method. We conclude with a brief description of Heritage Woods, a facility we see as the next significant development in facility care for the elderly and which we refer to as "the second generation Priory."

MEASURING SUCCESS

When the Priory programme was initiated, there were 71 women in various stages of mental and physical regression. The early results of the programme were evident in the statistics compiled by McIver after 11 months and are found in **Table 4.**

Table 4

Rewards of Remotivation

Activity	August, 1967	May, 1968
Eating in dining room	7%	90%
Confined to chair	87%	21%
Walking with aids	3%	28%
Self care	3%	20%
Socializing	5%	90%

McIver saw that there were also unintended consequences associated with a rehabilitation programme. As the residents improved some of them were re-classified and were no longer eligible for extended care. The Priory could no longer be their home as they had been led to believe. The residents saw that activation could mean discharge and it was not unknown that a family member would ask the administrator to stop all activities so that the person could re-main at the Priory. Those who could barely walk were still very fragile and dependent on good staff and friends. Without the support they would deterio-rate very quickly. McIver reports one situation in which a previously confused resident who was not able to walk improved and was able to be mobile using a walker. With the next assessment she was discharged to a Boarding Home. She didn't want to leave the Priory and in the new non-supportive environment she required heavy sedation and even restraints on occasion. She had a serious fall and was hospitalized. She was found to be dehydrated and had to have intravenous fluids. She would not tolerate this so restraints had to be applied. Three weeks later she was discharged back to the Priory but her recovery was poor. McIver asked if one would want to remotivate her again given these con-sequences?

While no formal programme evaluation was undertaken there were many indirect indicators of success. News of the Priory Method was spreading lo-cally, provincially, nationally and internationally. This was largely due to the fact that right from the start McIver spread the word about a new way to care for institutionalized elders. She did this through her articles, the skilled use of the media, workshops, speeches, presentations at conferences and by encouraging visitors and students to the site for a first-hand look and hands-on experience. Many of her written works are cited in the Reference List.

When the hospital became accredited in 1971 a footnote in the report read: "This hospital should be utilized educationally as much as possible, as a re-source example to other units."[74] That this advice did not fall on deaf ears can be seen from McIver's comments made at the Canadian Nurses Association convention in 1972. In that speech she publicly documented that members of all the health disciplines were coming to visit the Priory. She and her staff were giving lectures to baccalaureate and masters' nursing students. Visitors to the site included university professors. Some architects became interested in the Priory programme and as early as 1970 spent time at the Priory discussing resident's needs and observing the physical space. Copies of the film, *The Priory Method*, were in constant demand for nursing education and for staff inservice programmes within institutions. She told the convention that the recognition

---

[74]   McIver, V. (1972, June). <u>Rehabilitation of the Geriatric Patient</u>. Notes for a speech, CNA convention, Edmonton, Alberta. 4.

they were receiving showed the world what nursing power could do when it set its mind to improve care.

By 1973, six years of innovative changes in practice and management had transformed the face of health care at the Priory as well as affecting the practices of care staff in many agencies beyond its walls. For instance in April 1975 a delegation from the Alberta Hospital in Ponoka, Alberta visited the Priory. This hospital was a large institution primarily for mentally ill patients and included several wards of geriatric patients. Tony Karch, a member of the Faculty of Continuing Education at the University of Calgary, facilitated this visit. Karch went on to use his knowledge of the Priory Method in his Master's thesis, which proposed a psychosocial model for extended and long-term care facilities in Alberta. He was so enthusiastic about the Priory model of care that he organized workshops sponsored by the University, using Priory staff. [75]

In 1977, the hospital again received full accreditation. The hospital's efforts in providing high quality service to residents was recognized once more and it was seen to surpass the standards for providing good patient care. In addition, the style of administration was noted and commended as an example for others to follow.

EXPANSION OF THE ORGANIZATION

Up to the year 1973, St Mary's Priory in the House of Peace was the long-term care facility with a total of 71 residents under the leadership of Harrison and McIver. In 1973, the BC government purchased a 75-bed private hospital (Richmond Heights-Mt. Tolmie) and asked St. Mary's Priory administration under the Juan De Fuca Hospital Society Board of Directors to run the hospital. The decision was made to transfer the Priory organizational structure and management and care system to Mt. Tolmie. A Professional Services Coordinator and Unit Coordinator were appointed to manage the new unit. In February 1974, Glengarry Hospital (75 beds) was added, and in June 1975 Aberdeen Hospital (75 beds) was the final addition. This group eventually came to be known as the Juan de Fuca Hospitals. Each of the additional units was structured with the same management, staff positions and care programmes.

With the additional 225 residents, more professional and management staff were hired and shared amongst the hospitals. These included a Medical Coordinator, a Clinical Pharmacist, a Dietitian, a Physiotherapist, a Volunteer Coordinator, a Health Records Librarian and an Assistant Director of Health. These roles are elaborated on pages 76-77. In 1978 with the building of 150 new beds at

[75] Karch, A. J. (1980). A Psychosocial Model for Extended and Long-term Care Facilities in Alberta. Masters Thesis. University of Calgary. Calgary, Alberta.

Glengarry and 75 new beds at the Priory, a Director of Support Services was hired. During this expansion the staff from the Priory worked along side the staff in the new facilities to assist in the adoption of the philosophy and care model. As recorded in the report by Williamson:[76]

> The Priory organizational structure was used as a template for other extended care units. Other hospitals could institute a unit management structure based on the 75-bed unit principle. The health care services were multidisciplinary in nature under the direction of a Professional Services Coordinator with the Support Services [Hotel Management] supervised by the Unit Coordinators.

In order to enhance the contribution of the physician, a **Medical Coordinator** position was instituted. Physicians practicing in general practice and who had a particular interest and expertise in caring for the elderly filled this role. They were responsible for monitoring the attending physician's medical plan of care for each of a group of residents. They participated in the multidisciplinary resident review conferences and were involved in teaching staff.[77] Funding for these positions was obtained directly from the Medical Services Plan, Ministry of Health and provided for 4-hour weekly sessions for each 75-bed unit.[78]

The newly introduced roles took on a particular style consistent with the Restorative Care model. The **Clinical Pharmacist** had a clinical focus in addition to the packaging, dispensing and distribution of residents' medications. The clinical function ensured that the drugs being prescribed by the physician were appropriate therapy for the resident's condition and were monitored closely for side effects and drug interactions.[79] He served as a consultant to physicians on all drug issues. This became a critical role, as many drugs were not only ineffective but had dangerous side effects for the frail elderly.

The responsibilities of the **Clinical Dietitian** were expanded from providing nutritional assessments and care plans for residents. They now included menu planning, staff education on cultural and religious values which affected food likes and dislikes, preparation of a positive eating environment, organizing

---

[76] Williamson, F. (1978). An Environmental Study in Health Care: The Priory Concept and Extended Care Model: A Canadian Nursing Study Review. Unpublished monograph prepared as a result of a Florence Nightingale Scholarship. p6.

[77] Williamson, F. (1978). A Psychosocial Model of Health Care: The Priory Concept - a Baseline Approach: An Environment for Long-Term Care: A Canadian Nursing Study Review. Unpublished monograph prepared as a result of a Florence Nightingale Scholarship. 33.

[78] Juan De Fuca Hospital Society. (1977). Administrative Standards and Guidelines. Victoria, BC Unpublished.

[79] Williamson, F. (1978). An Environmental Study in Health Care: The Priory Concept and Extended Care Model: A Canadian Nursing Study Review. Unpublished monograph prepared as a result of a Florence Nightingale Scholarship. 64.

the special adaptive feeding utensils and the management of psychological aspects of eating.[80]

By the mid-seventies **Physiotherapists** were added to the team. Their responsibilities included a full resident assessment and they recommended a plan of care to the health team to ensure optimum physical and psychological functioning. In addition to their direct care function, they were responsible for in-service education on rehabilitation and therapeutic activation for staff. They were role models in demonstrating and supporting meaningful recreational and diversional activities for the residents.[81]

In addition to the standard responsibilities carried out in acute care, the **Health Records Librarian** was required to participate with the health care team to ensure that the resident's health record was complete and consistent with the concepts and philosophy of care. This was an important step in quality monitoring as it included assessing and evaluating the health record qualitatively on an ongoing basis. This was done to ensure that all necessary information was available to the health care team for the thorough assessment and care of the resident.[82]

To support the concept of community, a salaried **Volunteer Coordinator** position was initiated to recruit and support community volunteers who took on a major role in the psychosocial and spiritual component of care. These volunteer positions were not used as a substitute for professional staff but rather were a supplement to the resident care services, bringing the community life into the facility for the enjoyment of the resident.[83] The Volunteer Coordinator reporting to the PSC was responsible for the selection, orientation and supervision of volunteers. Volunteers were given resident-related activities consistent with their talents, training and experiences. Pastoral Care was one of the many programmes for which volunteers were recruited. The volunteer community clergy performed their duties as a part of the multidisciplinary team and provided one to one spiritual interactions, sacred music, bible reading, prayer and Sunday services.

The 1970 organizational chart was revised to reflect those changes shown above and is shown in **Figure 6** (on page 78).

---

[80] Williamson, F. 60.
[81] Williamson, F.. 58.
[82] Williamson, F. (1978). A Psychosocial Model of Health Care: The Priory Concept - a Baseline Approach: An Environment for Long-Term Care: A Canadian Nursing Study Review. Unpublished monograph prepared as a result of a Florence Nightingale Scholarship. 63.
[83] McIver, V. (1974, June 6). Total Involvement - A Challenge for Volunteers. Notes of a speech presented to the Canadian Hospitals' Convention. Vancouver, BC.

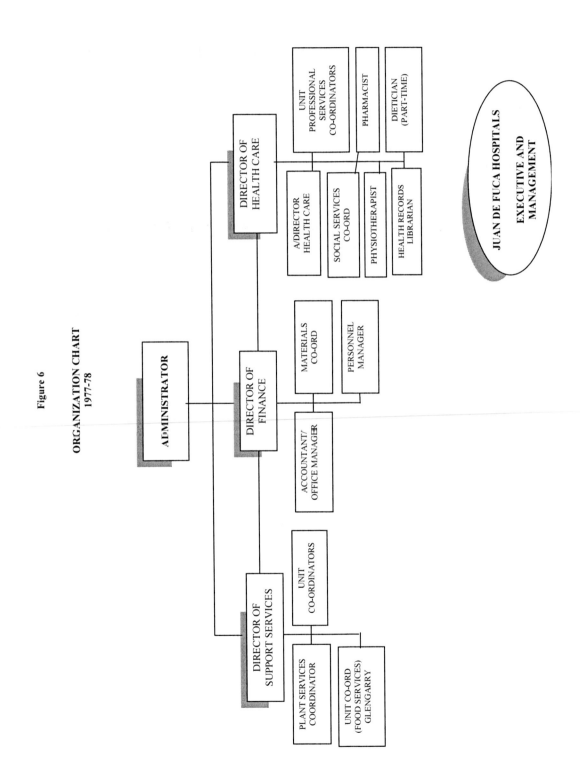

Figure 6

ORGANIZATION CHART
1977-78

THE EVOLUTION OF THE MODEL

By the time of McIver's retirement in 1979, the Priory Hospital had become one facility in the constellation of the four institutions known as the Juan de Fuca Hospitals. The term Priory continued as the name for the geographical site but the new hospital was called the Hiscock Unit after a former chairman of the Board. Many of the features of the Priory Method were embedded in the care practices of the staff in all the hospitals but by 1981 the term 'Priory Method' was no longer a term used by management and the majority of the staff.

Some of the basic components of the Restorative Care Model had undergone changes. For instance, the unit coordinator disappeared and a unit clerk with predominantly secretarial functions was in place. The term 'hotel services' was no longer in use. The numbers of professional disciplines other than nursing increased and there was a move to departmentalization. This was a trend McIver had rejected because she believed it focused more on the needs of the organization and the health professionals than on those of the resident. For her, direct accountability should remain with the manager closest to the resident and that was the Professional Services Coordinator. The non-nursing disciplines now reported to their department heads even though their assignments were unit-based and they maintained collaborative relationships with unit staff. The Professional Services Coordinator retained direct responsibility only for nursing and eventually the title of that position was changed to Director of Resident Care.

In McIver's day residents had stayed as long as 10-14 years at the Priory. This profile shifted because of alterations in the broader health care system such as the emergence of the provincial long-term care programme and the increase in home support services as well as changes in the profile of aging due to medical advances. By 1994 the length of stay had dropped to 1-2 years with many residents staying even shorter lengths of time before death.[84] Those residents who entered extended care had a much higher acuity level and approximately 80% had some degree of dementia, primarily of the Alzheimer type. Aggressive behaviors associated with declining cognitive status were increasing. The nature of the staff work changed and a much heavier workload ensued, as residents were frailer. New programmes such as the development of a dementia unit, respite care and a palliative care programme were brought on line to meet the changing resident needs. Care aides were now required to take a 20-week college-based programme to meet the need for better-trained staff but this usually did not include an explicit emphasis on the Priory Method.

---

[84]   Mantle, J. (1994). Resident Profile, Juan de Fuca Hospitals. Prepared by the Clinical Nurse Specialist Program.

Heritage Woods – The Second Generation Priory

In the nineties the Priory site itself underwent a significant change. There were no residents living in the original Priory Hospital but it did house a Day Programme and offered a service to about 30 seniors from the Western Communities. A new Director of Resident Care, Marilynne Convey, was appointed in 1993. Her most recent experience had been in community health and she had not encountered acute care practice for some years. Like McIver she had a wellness orientation. She was used to encountering clients in their home and saw the resident as the centre of the services.

Early in her tenure Convey was presented with the challenge of working with a team who would build a new facility for multilevel care on this site. In the end the site facilities would offer a broad spectrum of care, not dissimilar to the grand vision of Mother Cecelia in the 1950's. Three levels of care would be offered: extended care in the Hiscock facility; an adult day and community programme in a new building; and a new multilevel care facility with a focus on intermediate care called Heritage Woods. Intermediate Care was for those who were independently mobile but suffering from moderate to severe dementia or other chronic mental health problems and those who were physically frail but cognitively well.[85] Sudbury and Convey wrote about this project saying "Five years in the planning, this facility has the design, programming and staffing profile to make it one of the most unique in the country"[86] Consistent with the work of McIver, an old pattern of care was about to be broken and a new vision put forth. Themes from the past echoed anew but with a different flavor.

An extensive literature review (similar to the approach used by McIver in earlier years) was augmented by study visits on dementia care to Australia, Northern Europe, and within Canada. McIver's notion of creating a therapeutic community came to life again in a "design concept, staffing model and program chosen to maximize the capacity of the environment to act as a therapeutic tool."[87] One of the most important innovations was the replacement of the traditional, large group institution with 6 cottages each housing 12 or 13 residents.

---

[85]   Sudbury, F. and Convey, M. (2000, March). Facility design reflects latest dementia care concepts. Canadian Nursing Home. 11(1). 16.
[86]   Sudbury, Fiona and Convey, Marilynne (2000, March). 16.
[87]   Sudbury, Fiona and Convey, Marilynne (2000, March). 16.

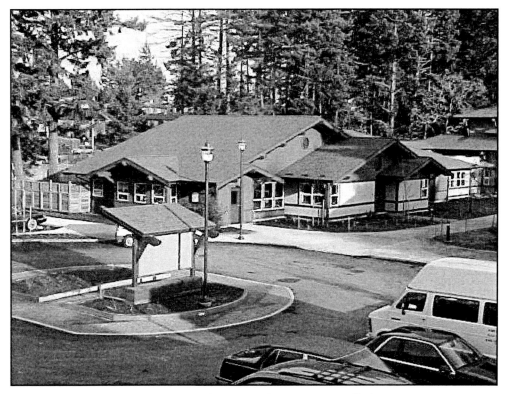

Heritage Woods, second generation Priory.

In this setting, home-like living becomes the order of the day as the residents are offered opportunities to participate in normal activities *in their own cottage*. Physical structural changes support the new model of care. Each cottage has its own fenced garden and a front entrance through which visitors enter just as one does at home. Administrative activities (reception, offices, staff room, hair dressing salon, two care centers, storage rooms and plant services) are located in a core that connects all the cottages but are not visible to the residents who live in the houses. This preserves the "home environment" and deinstitutionalizes the facility. Furniture, appliances, equipment and supplies are all non-institutional in appearance. Safety features are non-obtrusive as for example in having secondary shut-offs for the stove and oven and a lockable Dutch door to secure the kitchen. Just as in a home, socialization is fostered through the communal spaces of a cottage kitchen, a living room and a dining room as well as the garden. As with the Priory Method, activities occur in the communal area of each cottage and focus on meaningful social roles and familiar tasks.

As in McIver's time we see the introduction of new roles in order to achieve congruence with the model of care. The role of the Personal Care Attendant (PCA) was developed to provide both direct resident care and the enablement of residents in normal activities of daily living. The role is multifaceted as this staff person also does some laundry, food service and light housekeeping. Education for the role goes well beyond the usual preparation of Grade 10 schooling and the completion of the educational requirement for the Provincial Resident Care Attendant Programme. The PCA requires a Grade 12 education and completion of the provincial Resident Care Attendant Programme, the Activity Assistant Programme and the Food Safe Programme. The PCA focuses on maintaining the "person-hood" of the resident despite advancing cognitive impairment. "Being with" the resident, engendering trust and being a member of a team enhances their contribution to the therapeutic community.[88]

In a recent article Sudbury and Convey documented the values, the philosophy and the organization of care at Heritage Woods. In this facility the following ideas are valued: [89]

- The personality and previous lifestyle of each resident;
- Resident independence and freedom;
- Participation of family and friends in the lives of residents;
- The unique contribution of staff;
- The importance of reaching out to the community;
- The contribution that research makes in improving care.

In discussing the philosophy and organization of care they write that:[90]

- Heritage Woods staff work co-operatively as a team that also includes residents, family, friends and volunteers.
- The focus of daily life is to enable residents to participate in normal daily activities such as self-care, grooming and dressing, bed-making, meal preparation/cooking, cleaning/dusting, laundry, leisure and recreation, gardening, exercise and games.
- It is recognized that memories are a resident's most precious possession; as such, efforts are made to promote reminiscence through familiar activities.
- The creation of a caring and therapeutic environment where residents feels safe, respected and important, requires a partnership and helping relationship between resident, family, staff and volunteers. This care methodology also requires that staff understand

[88]   Sudbury, F. and Convey, M. (2000, March). Facility design reflects latest dementia care concepts. Canadian Nursing Home. 11(1). 17.
[89]   Sudbury, F. and Convey, M. (2000, March). 21.
[90]   Sudbury, F. and Convey, M. (2000, March). 21.

the therapeutic use of self, which means that staff act as role models for residents, using a calm and respectful manner in their interactions.

- Regular staff are assigned in a manner that utilizes their unique skills and abilities, and promotes continuity of care.

These values, philosophy, and ways of organizing care speak both to the durability of the earlier messages of McIver whilst reflecting advances in caring for persons in long term care. Heritage Woods is another milestone in the history of resident-centered caring. It reflects, once again, the imaginative nursing leadership that emerges from time to time. From these creative endeavors we humbly draw our guidance and inspiration to go forward.

Reference List

Alsop, K. (1971, December 9, 10, 11). A Miracle from Great Expectations, Therapy of Doing, Mind comes First. A 3 part series. The Province. Vancouver, BC.

Argyris, C. (1957). Personality and Organization. New York: Harper and Row.

Bambiger, B., Milord, J. (Eds.). (1975). Gifts of Aging: An Anthology of the Human Journey. Victoria: Unpublished.

Baum, D J. (1977). Warehouses for Death: The Nursing Home Industry. Ontario: Burns & MacEachern Limited.

BCNU demands changes to non-nursing work and overtime abuse. Times Colonist. (2001, May). Victoria, BC.

Birren, T. (1970). Color for Interiors-Historical and Modern. New York: Whitney Publications Inc.

Braddock, J. (1973, February 27). Hospital walls should be ripped down. The Province. Vancouver, BC.

Corbett, T. L. & Lai, D. M. (1979). Searching for euthanatos: the hospice alternative. Hospital Progress. 60(3). 38-41, 76.

Dombowsky, Sister Mary Elizabeth (2001). Personal Conversations. Victoria, BC.

Dunsmuir, R (1973, April). Seniors gain fuller lives when wards lose starch. The Colonist. Victoria, BC.

Elderly enjoy new life thanks to good citizen. (1969, June 8). Daily Colonist. Victoria, BC.

Forbes, W. F., Jackson, J. F., & Kraus, A. S. (1987). Institutionalization of the Elderly in Canada. Toronto: Butterworths.

Gain, D. (1968, April 4). Patients find new goals. Daily Colonist. Victoria, BC.

Hertzberg, H. (1966). Work and the Nature of Man. Montreal: Crowell Press.

Juan De Fuca Hospital Society. (1977). Administrative Standards and Guidelines. Victoria, BC. Unpublished.

Juan De Fuca Hospital Society. (1977). Educational Manual. Victoria. BC. Unpublished.

Karch, A. J. (1980). A Psychosocial Model for Extended and Long-term Care Facilities in Alberta. Masters Thesis. University of Calgary. Calgary, Alta.

Likert, R. (1967). Human Organization. Toronto: McGraw Hill.

Mantle, J. (1994). Unpublished teaching notes. University of Victoria. Victoria, BC.

Mantle, J. (1994). Resident Profile Juan De Fuca Hospitals. Prepared by CNS Program. Victoria, BC.

Mantle, J. (2003). Analysis of the Tree Drawings. Victoria, BC.

McIver V. (Producer). (1968). Priory Method Film. Silent film shot on color Super 8 camera. Victoria, BC.

McIver, V. (Producer). (1968). The Priory Method - Extended Care - Remotivation. Videotape made from a 16 mm Movie Film. Juan de Fuca Hospitals, Victoria, BC.

McIver, V. (1969, April). Communal dining. Canadian Nurse Journal. 65 (4). 6.

McIver, V. (1970, June). St Mary's Priory Job Description for Care Coordinators. Unpublished paper. Victoria, BC.

McIver, V. (1970, August). Creative Chronic Care-the Priory Method. Vancouver Island Catholic News. 2 (6), 8-9.

McIver, V. (1970). How the social worker can fit into our picture. Unpublished paper.

McIver, V. (1971, Aug 19). Acute Care Philosophy Versus Extended Care Philosophy. A speech presented at Malaspina College, Nanaimo, BC.

McIver, V. (1971, August). The role of the RN in extended care. Unpublished paper.

McIver, V (1971, July). Reap your own harvest. Unpublished paper.

McIver, V. (1971). Workload staff requirements. Unpublished paper.

McIver, V. (1972, January 19). Focus On Aging. Notes for a paper presentation at the Interprofessional Course, University of British Columbia, Vancouver, BC.

McIver V. (1972, December). For a more human approach to long-term patient care Hospital Administration in Canada. 55-57

McIver, V. (1972). Rehabilitation of the Geriatric Patient. Notes for a speech at CNA Convention, Edmonton, Alta.

McIver, V. (1972, November). Staffing. Paper given to The Registered Nurses Association of British Columbia. Vancouver, BC.

McIver, V. (1973, February). A New Environment for Extended Care. Proceedings of the Seminar on Extended Care. British Columbia Hospitals' Association. Richmond, BC.

McIver, V. (1974). <u>Total Involvement – A Challenge for Volunteers</u>. Notes of a speech presented to the Canadian Hospitals' Convention, Vancouver, BC.

McIver, V. (1974, July). Notes for presentation to staff at Ponoka Long Term Care Facility, Ponoka, Alberta.

McIver, V. (1974, September). <u>Reactivation to Self-Feeding</u>. Paper presented at The Priory Hospital, Victoria, BC.

McIver, V. (1974, October 1). <u>Policies Were Meant to be Broken</u>. Notes for a speech presented at the Long-term Care Conference. Geneva Park, Lake Couchiching, Ont.

McIver, V. (1975, April). <u>I Am a Unique Person</u> Notes of a speech presented at the Saskatchewan Association of Special Care Homes Convention. Saskatoon, Sask.

McIver, V. (1976, March 26). <u>Cast Me Not Off in the Time of My Death</u>. Speech presented at St. Joseph's School of Nursing. Victoria, BC.

McIver, V. (1976, November). <u>With Dignity and Respect</u>. Notes of a speech given at the University of Victoria, Victoria, BC.

McIver, V. (1977, July). <u>Humanizing the workplace.</u> Unpublished paper. Victoria, BC.

McIver, V. (1978, March 25). Freedom to be: A new approach to quality care for the aged. <u>Canadian Nurse Journal. 74 (3) 19-25</u>

McIver, V. (1979, November). Organization of integrated extended care facilities. <u>Dimensions in Health Care</u>. 20-23.

McIver, V. (1980, September). A time to be born: a time to die. <u>The Canadian Nurse</u>. <u>76</u> (8). 38-41.

McIver, V. (1999). Unpublished manuscript. Victoria, BC.

McIver, V. (2000, 2001, 2002). Personal Interviews. Victoria, BC.

Narroway, M. D. (December, 1974). <u>Living Message</u>. 6.

National Film Board of Canada. (Producer). (1979). <u>The Priory: The only Home I've Got</u>. Ottawa, Ont.

Saunders, P. (1976). Lesson 12, Section IV: Specific Implementation of Concepts. <u>Programme Manual</u>. Unpublished.

Saunders, P. (1976). Lesson 13, Section III Remotivation Therapy – What is it? <u>Programme Manual</u>. Unpublished.

Sudbury, F., Convey, M. (2000, March,). Facility design reflects latest dementia care concepts. <u>Canadian Nursing Home</u>, <u>11</u> (1). 16 - 21.

St. Mary's Priory Hospital. (1970, June). Job Description. Care Coordinator. Unpublished.

Vipond, D. (1975, January 14). Home movies become real thing. A time to rejoin the living. Victoria Times. Victoria, BC.

Vipond, D. (1975, April 5). St Mary's Priory admired. Victoria Times. Victoria, BC.

Warick, R. (1972, June 20). Patients emotional needs stressed. Leader Post. Regina, Sask

We can do more. (1968, October 16). Juan De Fuca News-Review. Colwood, BC.

Williamson, F. (1978). A Psychosocial Model of Health Care: The Priory Concept - a Baseline Approach: An Environment for Long-Term Care: A Canadian Nursing Study Review. Unpublished monograph prepared as a result of a Florence Nightingale Scholarship. England.

Williamson, F. (1978). An Environmental Study In Health Care. The Priory Concept. An Extended Care Module. A Canadian Nursing Study Review. Unpublished monograph prepared as a result of a Florence Nightingale Scholarship. England.

Wing, D. (2003). Adapted from McIver, V., Patrick, G., & Dolny, J. (1972, June). Custodial Care Tree. Unpublished drawing. Victoria, BC.

Wing, D. (2003). Adapted from McIver, V., Patrick, G., & Dolny, J. (1972, June). Restorative Care Tree. Unpublished drawing. Victoria, BC.

Significant Dates in the Development of the Priory Method

1951   · Mother Cecelia bought the clubhouse of the Royal Colwood Golf Course.
       Architects were asked to renovate the clubhouse into a convent and
       space for a care facility for elderly ladies. Mother scrapped the project
       because of revisions required by BCHIS.
       · Mother Cecelia renovated the building herself using day labor and
       making spaces for 49 patients recovering from sickness and for elderly
       ladies. She called it the *Priory Convalescent Home*.

1953   · The restaurant on this Golf Course property, Chez Marcel, was con-
       verted into a care facility for 24 patients. Mother called it the Hospital
       but it was a home for older ladies

1954   · Mother built the *House of Peace* and admitted 50 severely impaired
       patients. It was blessed by the bishop in November 1956 and often housed
       about 100 patients.
       · The caretaker's house on the property was converted into a medical
       and dental centre with an x-ray department.
       · A laundry was established in the tool shed and served the complexes
       as well as neighbouring motels.

1957   · Mother Cecelia purchased the Royal Auto Court directly across the
       street. It had 16 units and a large house. It was called the *"City of Peace"*.
       She now had a full range of care from rest home patients to extended
       care but the quality of care was in question.

1962   · Mother Cecelia left the Colwood properties and lost control of the
       operation of the Sisters of the Love of Jesus

1966   · BCHIS takes over the little hospital of 24 beds as an Extended Care
       Unit for which they would pay all expenses
       · An Advisory board was formed to assist the Priory Sisters

1967   · Feb 1 House of Peace accepted as Extended Care Unit - Opened Octo-
       ber 5, 1967
       · 90 beds were reduced to 71
       · Renovations were undertaken by Bragg and Hamilton, architects

1967   · April 1 appointments
           George Harrison - Administrator & Comptroller
           Vera McIver as Nursing Director

1967   · McIver begins correspondence courses with American Catholic Hospital
       Association

1967   · October 5 – Opening of the renovated House of Peace

1968   · March 6th -Workshop at the Priory on Rehabilitation of the Old Frail given by Sister Laurice Baudry OSB from Minnesota. BCHIS invited as well as extended care hospitals in the region. Talk included a discussion on Reactivation

1968 · Pet therapy started
· February 5, 1968 First issue of Spectrum, a monthly bulletin was published. This was both an informational update about people and events as well as a vehicle for in-service. McIver's articles in this bulletin were included in the BCHIS bulletin beginning in late 1968 and were continued for some time.

1969 · McIver studied Canadian Nurses Association course in Nursing Administration

1970 · McIver started 2-year Hospital Organization and Management correspondence course sponsored by the Canadian Hospital Association in collaboration with the University of Manitoba. (Ended in 1972)
· This led to membership in the Canadian College of Health Service Executives as well as Provincial Administrator Associations

1971 · Accreditation awarded in September

1973 · Mt Tolmie Hospital added
· January – First social worker hired at Priory Hospital

1974 · Glengarry Hospital (75 beds) and Aberdeen Hospital (75 beds) added to the complex

1975 · Juan de Fuca Society officially took over the two Priory Hospitals·
Peggy Saunders hired as Assistant to McIver and played a major inservice role
· April – delegation from Ponoka hospital, Alberta made their first visit to the Priory

1977 · All 4 units accredited

1978 · September – CEO George Harrison left

1978 · Band participated in Lions Telethon
· Medical Advisory Committee became active

1978 · Elizabeth Laugharne hired as Assistant to McIver

1979 · January - Glengarry expansion opened
· February - Jack Howard hired to fill the position of CEO
· July - New beds opened at the Priory Hiscock unit
· Dental Survey
· National Film Board released film "The Priory: The Only Home I've Got"

1979 · March – retirement of McIver

1986 · McIver received The Order of Canada Award

ISBN 1553957490